CHALLENGING MEDICAL ETHICS

Volume 1

No Water – No Life:
Hydration in the Dying

CHALLENGING MEDICAL ETHICS.
Volume 1 No Water – No Life: Hydration in the Dying

ISBN 0 9545445 3 6

Please address orders and enquiries about this book to:
PO Box 341, Enterprise House, NORTHAMPTON NN3 2WZ, UK
or e-mail: books 341 @clara.co.uk for further information.

This book has been compiled to increase understanding of a
controversial and sensitive aspect of medical practice. The publisher,
editor and distributors can take no responsibility for any actions or
omissions that result from the content of this publication, or of any
references cited therein. The views expressed are those of individual
authors with widely differing opinions. All doctors and nurses have
a responsibility to respect human life, and should at all times act in
their patient's best interest.

Fairway Folio
(Christian Publishing Services)
Alsager, Cheshire, UK
Tel: 01270 874662

Printed by Pegasus Print Ltd, Northampton, UK

No Water – No Life:
Hydration in the Dying

Compiled and edited by Gillian Craig

This book charts a decade of debate about the ethical provision of hydration in the terminally ill and dying. This is an extremely controversial and sensitive area of medical practice that has serious implications for countless patients and their relatives. The spotlight falls on a regime of sedation without hydration that is sometimes used at the end of life. The question at issue is "Has palliative medicine gone too far?" Those who question received wisdom are too easily silenced. This book gives them a voice.

**"Disagreement is essential and fundamental
to the way science works."**

Professor Colin Blakemore

Acknowledgements

I thank all the people who have contributed to the debate, including Professor R. Gillon, when Editor of the *Journal of Medical Ethics*, many senior people in public life, colleagues in palliative medicine, and members of the public who share my concerns. The Royal College of Physicians of London and the Centre for Bioethics and Public Policy organised platforms for debate in London.

I am indebted to the following publishers for permission to reprint their copyright material:-

- BMJ Publishing Group for articles from the *Journal of Medical Ethics.*

- The Centre for Bioethics and Public Policy for an article from *Ethics and Medicine.*

- *Hayward Medical* Communications for extracts from the *European Journal of Palliative Care (1997).*

- *The British Journal of Hospital Medicine (1986)* for extracts from an article by Twycross.

- *Hospital Medicine* (2000)-for use of a table by Jackson.

- The National Council for Hospice and Specialist Palliative Care Services for permission to print their guidelines of July/August 1997.

- *The Medico-Legal Journal* (1994) for an article by Craig.

- The Medical Defence Union, London for extracts from an article by Turner.

- Prime National Publishing Corp. 470 Boston Post Road, Weston MA 02493 for an article by Baumrucher from the *American Journal of Hospice and Palliative Care.*1999; 16: 502-3 and quotes from an article by Morita et al. in the same volume.

- *Springer-Verlag* for permission to use copyright figures on pages 96 and 97.

- *Fortress Press Philadelphia* for quotes from 'Politics Medicine & Christian Ethics.' 1973.

- International Society of Nephrology for use of their copyright figure on p. 97.

- The General Medical Council for quotes from their guidance of August 2002.

Contributors

The following people made contributions to the debate:-

Professor Michael Ashby, Monash University, Victoria, Australia.

Dr M J Baines, Consultant Physician, St Christoper's Hospice, London, UK.

Dr Steven Baumrucker, Medical Director, Housecall Hospice, Tennessee, USA.

Professor Eduardo Bruera and colleagues in Edmonton, Alberta, Canada.

Dr Anthony Cole, Founder of the Medical Ethics Alliance.

Dr Gillian Craig, retired Consultant Geriatrician, Northampton, UK.

C. Docker. Director of Exit, Edinburgh, Scotland.

Professor R Downie, Professor of Moral Philosophy, Glasgow.

Dr R Dunlop, formerly Medical Director, St. Christopher's Hospice.

Dr Kilian Dunphy, Chaired Ethics Committee. Association for Palliative Medicine (APM) of Great Britain and Ireland. Debated issues with Craig at Royal College of Physicians in 1997.

Dr J Ellershaw, Medical Director, Liverpool Marie Curie Centre.

Dr Robin L Fainsinger of Canada working with Professor Eduardo Bruera and colleagues.

Professor Ilora Finlay, Cardiff, who chaired Ethics Committee APM of GB & Ireland, in 1994.

Dr James Gilbert, Consultant Physician in Palliative Medicine, Exeter, UK.

Professor Raanan Gillon of Imperial College, London, formerly editor of the Journal of Medical Ethics.

Dr Fiona Hicks, when Senior Registrar, Wheatfields Hospice, Leeds.

Dr L Hepburn, Director, Provincial Bioethics Centre, Queensland, Australia.

Dr Maurice A Jackson, Consultant Physician and Nephrologist, Wolverhampton, UK.

Dr T Morita and colleagues in Japan.

Dr Fiona Randall. Chaired Joint Working Party preparing guidelines.

Dr Gillian Rathbone. Consultant, Ashby-de-la-Zouch, UK.

Dame Cicely Saunders, Hon. President of The National Council for Hospice & Specialist Palliative Care Services. (NCHSPCS) of London.

Dr Brian Stoffell, Director, Medical Ethics Unit, Flinders University of South Australia.

Professor Margaret Somerville, Centre for Medical Ethics and Law, McGill University, Canada.

Dr N Sykes, Consultant Physician, now Medical Director of St Christopher's Hospice.

Dr Robert Twycross. Reader in Palliative Medicine Oxford University and Hon. Consultant Physician, Sir Michael Sobell House, Oxford.

Nancy Guilfoy Valko. Author and Registered Nurse of California, USA.

Dr Eric Wilkes, Consultant Adviser to Trent Palliative Care Centre, UK.

The Editor

Dr Gillian Craig MD, FRCP

Qualified at St Thomas's Hospital Medical School, London University, and subsequently worked in the Departments of Medicine at the University of Cambridge and Birmingham, England. She studied aspects of renal physiology as a Research Assistant at Cambridge, and neuroendocrinology as a Visiting Scientist in Massachusetts. The final years of a varied medical career were spent as a Consultant Geriatrician in Northampton. Since retirement from clinical practice in 1993 she has written papers on medical ethics and other issues that concern her.

Contents

Introduction

Palliative care is a relatively new but rapidly expanding branch of medicine that was given specialty status in the UK in 1987. The specialty as defined by the World Health Organisation in 1990 is, in essence "The active and total care of patients whose disease is not responsive to curative treatment. Control of pain and other symptoms, and of psychological, social and spiritual problems is paramount...". Most of the patients who are cared for in hospices have terminal cancer, but some are in the terminal stages of other conditions such as motor neurone disease or AIDS. When death is inevitable and imminent as a consequence of incurable disease, control of pain and other symptoms becomes the aim, rather than prolongation of life at all costs. Nevertheless intentional shortening of life should be prohibited and all reasonable measures that enhance the comfort of the patient should be employed.

This book is about the value of hydration in the care of the dying. The difficult question of the use of sedation without hydration is explored. Some see this as an effective way of controlling severe symptoms at the end of life; others view it as a covert form of euthanasia. Palliative carers are naturally keen to distance themselves from any such suggestion, but the criticism is a valid one that cannot be dismissed. In law a doctor can give treatment that may shorten life, provided that the intention is to relieve pain or other distressing symptoms in the dying. This traditional line of defence, known as the doctrine of double effect, protects doctors from unjustified accusations of murder, but is also open to abuse. The doctrine is now under close scrutiny by the legal profession.

I raised concerns about a regime of sedation without hydration with senior members of the medical profession in 1990 and was invited to write a paper for the Journal of Medical Ethics. Publication of this paper in 1994 provoked wide debate. Behind the scenes in the United Kingdom committees were convened to draw up guidelines on the ethical use of artificial hydration in terminally ill patients, which were published by the National Council for Hospice and Specialist Palliative Care Services in 1997. Opinion was deeply divided between those who favoured the use of hydration in the dying and those who did not. Some felt that my criticism had struck at the whole ethos of palliative medicine. The ethical and legal issues raised by the hydration debate proved to be extremely complex. This book documents a decade of debate.

Contributions to the debate were published in the Journal of Medical Ethics, the Medico-Legal Journal, Ethics and Medicine, Palliative Medicine, the European Journal of Palliative Care, the American Journal of Hospice and Palliative Care, the Journal of Pain and Symptom Management, the Catholic Medical Quarterly and the Journal of Terminal Oncology between 1994 and 2003. I have included several key papers in this book to create an historical record of the debate in a readily accessible form. Others that are equally important, but perhaps rather too medical for a general reader have been omitted. My aim has been to present the debate in the words of the main protagonists, and to show the public how the medical profession deals with dissent. The book is a collage, an anthology, a collection of papers and comments- a long conversation about the importance of hydration in the care of the dying.

Informed debate about medical matters is hard to achieve in the public sphere, but through articles in major newspapers in the UK, occasional documentary reports on television, and in some cases painful personal experience, many people have caught a glimpse of the problems that can arise in our hospitals and hospices. Sadly the hydration debate has become a battleground for advocates and opponents of voluntary euthanasia, for the former are quick to suggest that a lethal injection might be preferable to a lingering death from dehydration. Thus it is vital that palliative carers heed this danger and pay attention to the need for hydration at the end of life.

I have included some case reports to illustrate the sort of problems that can arise at the end of life. It is sometimes easier to understand ethical dilemmas when illustrated by case reports, than when discussed in impersonal generalities. Every patient is different and the correct course of action must take account of all aspects of their case. For reasons of confidentiality the identity of the patients and relatives cannot be revealed, unless the information is already in the public sphere. Readers may find some of the case reports disturbing, but every sphere of human activity has its dark side. Progress can only be made when darkness is acknowledged and overcome.

During the course of the hydration debate I have been encouraged and helped by people too numerous to mention, but particular thanks must go to Professor Raanan Gillon, former Editor of the Journal of Medical Ethics, whose interest and support in the early years of the debate was invaluable. To all who have contributed to the debate in any way, by replying to letters, sending me newspaper articles, typing the manuscript, allowing me to use copyright material, publishing my papers, responding to my criticism and taking the debate forward, I send my warm thanks. Through my interest in medical ethics I have been privileged to know some brave and determined people who are struggling to be heard in a culture of concealment. I pay tribute to them and hope that my work will prove helpful to them.

Dr Gillian Craig

Chapter 1

Setting The Scene

"Disagreement is essential and fundamental
to the way science works."
Professor Colin Blakemore

Author Gillian Craig

When I qualified as a doctor in London in 1963, palliative care did not exist as a specialty, and Paul Ramsay had not formulated his influential ideas about care, and care only, for the dying. But for a painful personal experience in 1990 I might be blissfully ignorant about "comfort care" to this day. Fate had a different plan for me, for I found myself in the role of a visitor at a hospice and discovered that hospice staff were quite prepared to sedate a patient and to continue sedation, without hydration, for days on end, until the patient died in a grossly dehydrated state. In one particularly disturbing case I felt that I had witnessed a slow form of euthanasia. I was appalled.

Coming from a background of hospital medicine I felt strongly that hydration should be maintained by the use of a drip if need be, in order to prevent death from dehydration. The hospice doctor on the other hand felt equally strongly that some patients should be allowed to die. Gross dehydration did not bother her and drips were anathema to her, for in her view they merely prolonged the dying process. The ideological gap between us could not be bridged. Both of us cared for dying patients in the course of our work but our approach was entirely different.

As a Consultant Geriatrician, I had a life-supportive, treatment-orientated approach to a dying patient. As a Palliative Care Physician, the hospice doctor had a death-orientated approach. Who was right? Is hydration a basic human need? If so, how can it be morally right for a doctor to withhold hydration from a dying patient? These are just some of the questions that are addressed in the hydration debate.

I left that hospice resolved to do whatever I could to put an end to the practice of terminal sedation. In due course there was an inquiry into the management of the case I had witnessed, but two independent palliative care consultants supported their colleague, taking the view that the case had been handled professionally and well. Clearly there was a need for wide debate of the ethical issues that loomed so large in my mind, and so the hydration debate was born.

Many people view the hospice movement through rose-tinted spectacles, but it has its darker side. As in any human institution, nothing is perfect and attitudes can become rather rigid. Death can become rather insistent in a hospice -almost obligatory - for the aim of the staff is to ensure that the patients have a 'good death'.[1] The provision of fluids by means of a drip may be opposed by some hospice doctors who, like the one I encountered, argue that drips simply prolong dying. Treatment-orientated doctors feel equally strongly that fluid should be provided, by a drip if need be, as this prolongs life, prevents dehydration and may make the patient more comfortable. Hospice staff do all that they can to ensure that death, when it comes, will be peaceful.

Stories of great compassion and gentleness abound, but as W H Auden wrote in his poem 'First things first' - "Thousands have lived without love, not one without water." [2]

Technology is accepted in a hospice if it is needed for pain or symptom control, but to use technology merely to prolong life is frowned upon for it prolongs the dying process. Thus the use of drips to maintain hydration may be viewed with great suspicion. Drips are considered 'intrusive' by palliative carers, they are said to interfere with the dignity of death and are seen as a potential barrier between patients and loved ones. On the other hand, syringe pumps used to deliver powerful sedatives and pain killers -even tubes inserted into the spinal canal for pain relief, are regarded as acceptable. It makes little sense. Clearly technology itself is not the problem, it all depends on the use to which technology is put. Technology for symptom control is acceptable in a hospice, but technology used to prolong life is resented. It is as simple as that. Thus the level of care that a patient receives will depend to a large extent on the setting. Patients dying at home or in a hospice or nursing home are far less likely to have a drip than patients dying in a hospital ward. In 1990 a drip was almost unheard of in a hospice. Dehydration was considered to be a normal part of the dying process and to do anything to prevent it was 'meddlesome'. On the other hand, on hospital wards at that time drips were used very frequently - no one thought twice about it, if the patient was dehydrated you put up a drip - to have done otherwise would have been considered wrong.

Attitudes to hydration in the hospice movement began to change in the early 1990's. Fainsinger and Bruera reported the use of hypodermoclysis i.e. a subcutaneous infusion of fluid for symptom control in 1991,[3] and later in 1994 they reported the use of this technique for rehydration in terminally ill patients.[4] However, for some reason their work has not been greeted with great enthusiasm in the United Kingdom where a more traditional approach is favoured. My personal role in the hydration debate has been to highlight the ethical, legal and medical dangers of a regime of sedation without hydration in the dying and to draw attention to the plight of dissenting relatives. Much has been achieved in the last decade, for attitudes to hydration in the hospice movement in the United Kingdom have become more flexible thanks to the constructive response of colleagues to my criticism. There are now two schools of thought about hydration in palliative care. Some doctors would use a drip to prevent dehydration in the dying, but others would not. A hard core of traditional hospice doctors view the changing attitudes to hydration with concern and do their best to thwart them, for the hospice movement was started by Dame Cicely Saunders partly to shield people from inappropriate attempts to prolong life. In the United Kingdom much palliative medicine is undertaken in the community by general practitioners (GPs) with and without Consultant advice. Many hospices are supported by GP clinical assistants and many GP trainees are exposed to hospice philosophy in their formative years. Inflexible non-interventionist attitudes to hydration in the dying may therefore be prevalent in the wider community.

The 'management of death' has moved centre stage in recent years, especially in the USA where economists and politicians seek to contain health-care costs. Where America leads other nations tend to follow. The tendency now in the USA and in Great Britain, is for doctors to withhold and withdraw life-prolonging medical treatment from dying or severely debilitated patients, such as elderly people with severe strokes or dementia. Medical ethics has become polluted by politics!

It is undoubtedly true that some doctors are guilty of using technology too much. The syndrome is described by cynics as "never give up ethics".[5] The art of medicine is to know when to treat and use technology to preserve and sustain life, and when to refrain from futile intervention. There is however, a narrow demarcation line between withholding treatment and causing death by negligence. Quite a considerable volume of literature relates to the borderland between killing and letting die.[6,7]

The spectrum of medical care

Attitudes to technological intervention and life support in medicine fall, broadly speaking, into three groups as shown in Figure 1. The spectrum extends from intensive life support on the one hand - if there is the remotest chance of recovery, through a middle ground, to a death-orientated approach, when technology is used for the patient's comfort but not to prolong life.

Intensive life-support includes intensive care, mechanical ventilation, renal dialysis, heart transplants and other forms of heroic surgery. The "never say die" practitioners may be found at this end of the spectrum. Here you may find patients with severe heart failure and lung failure waiting for life-saving transplants. Here also you will find accident victims, and others who if treated actively may make a full recovery.

In the middle ground you will find most general medical and surgical wards, and geriatric rehabilitation wards in the hospital sector. Here, patients with strokes and other common illnesses, including cancer in the early and treatable stage, are cared for and actively treated. Artificial hydration and nutrition will be used as and when necessary to support life, until such time as a recovery occurs or the patient dies. Death from dehydration or starvation on these wards should give cause for concern.

On the left of the spectrum is palliative care. The word palliative is derived from the Latin 'pallium' which means to cloak or hide, for symptoms are cloaked and hidden. Most palliative care doctors regard themselves as life-affirming and are opposed to euthanasia. They accept the inevitability of death and do nothing to hasten or postpone the dying process. Prolonged sedation without hydration falls in a legal grey area. There are grounds for saying that it is tantamount to euthanasia at times but this has not yet been tested in court. Its use should be reserved for those whose symptoms and distress cannot be controlled in any other way. The ethical and legal problems associated with the use of sedation without hydration are explored in this book.

Figure 1
The spectrum of medical care

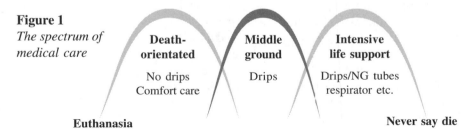

Death-orientated	Middle ground	Intensive life support
No drips Comfort care	Drips	Drips/NG tubes respirator etc.

Euthanasia   **Never say die**

3

On the extreme left of the spectrum are those who campaign for euthanasia or doctor assisted suicide. Euthanasia is better described as murder, for that is what it is. Some people favour a lethal injection as a means of ending life, but in most countries of the world such an action is illegal.

An historical perspective

The ethical problems created by prolonged sedation without hydration in terminal care received little attention prior to publication of my paper in the Journal of Medical Ethics in 1994.[8] In an earlier discussion paper from the USA published in the New England Journal of Medicine in 1992 the authors discussed the use of barbiturates in the care of the terminally ill, on the basis of four case reports. No mention was made of the need for hydration since most of the patients died within two days of sedation.[9]

A paper from the Netherlands, published in 1999 described the use of sedation in two hospice patients, but the issue of hydration was not mentioned. The authors took the conventional view that life-prolonging treatment is "potentially harmful for the well-being of terminal patients . . .", since it can make acceptance of their situation more difficult, and is "futile". Nevertheless they considered that hastening death is "dangerous and unnecessary"[10] . . . a view with which I heartily agree! The authors were writing in the context of euthanasia by lethal injection as practised in the Netherlands. It is strange that palliative carers still find it difficult to accept that withholding life-prolonging treatment, including hydration, is sometimes equivalent to shortening life. The hydration debate is as relevant now as it was in the 1990s!

A theological perspective

The origins of conventional thinking on the care of the dying can be traced to the work of Paul Ramsay, an influential theologian, writing around 1970.[11] Ramsay developed a theology of care, and only care, for the dying. My understanding of his work is based on a book by Charles Curran entitled 'Politics, Medicine and Christian Ethics' that was published in 1973.[12]

Curran wrote - "The distinction between the use of ordinary and extraordinary means to preserve life is related to two other important distinctions - the distinction between saving life and prolonging dying, as well as the distinction between direct killing and allowing the patient to die...An ethic of only caring for the dying is opposed to two extremes: the one that affirms there is never any reason not to use or to stop using all available means to preserve life, and the other extreme which justifies positive euthanasia or the direct taking of the life of a terminal patient . . . Ramsay argues that not using or withdrawing extraordinary means is not merely doing nothing, but rather can be positively called part of our care for, and accompanying of, the person in his dying . . . Ramsay argues that the Christian theology of care means that one attend the dying patient and not unnecessarily prolong dying."[12]

Karl Barth insisted on the sanctity of life and 'ruled out any pettifogging distinction between directly killing and allowing to die, but conceded that a doctor might have to recoil from a prolongation of life which would be the equivalent of human arrogance in the face of impending death'.[13] Ramsay accepted the view of Gerald Kelly 'who described the ordinary means of preserving life as those medicines, treatments and operations which offer a reasonable hope of benefit for the patient, and which can be obtained and used without excessive pain, expense or other inconvenience'.[14]

Theologians in the 1970's and earlier, recognised that 'there are broader, non-medical reasons which make certain treatments elective. In these cases the doctor acts more as a man (or woman!) than as a medical expert. There is (said Ramsay) a difference between the medical and the moral imperative, but they are not separable in the person, or in the vocation of a person who is a physician'.[12]

Many people argue that once the dying process has begun, or "irreversibly encompassed the person" our relationship to that person and his/her claims upon us change.[12] However it can be extremely difficult to distinguish those who are irretrievably dying, from those who are apparently dying, but whose situation is reversible with active and good medical care. To withhold treatment, including hydration from patients who are not irreversibly dying, will render their condition fatal. It is far safer in medical terms, to err in favour of life. A person who is irretrievably dying will die regardless of medical intervention, and treatment may indeed be futile. However quietly supporting life with artificial hydration can achieve surprising and rewarding results, and may add to the overall comfort of the patient.

I question the long established and conventional approach to the care of the dying. The hydration debate raises important questions about the whole ethos of palliative care. I question whether simple forms of artificial hydration can be regarded as extraordinary means of prolonging life. If one accepts the views of Kelly, such measures must be regarded as ordinary. In terms of other aspects of medical technology, such as renal dialysis and heart transplants, a subcutaneous infusion is very ordinary and mundane. The question then arises as to whether maintaining physiological equilibrium and biological life is of benefit to the patient. Such questions introduce the concept of the value of life, and whether this can be quantified. Those who regard human life as sacred under all circumstances hold one view, those who regard human life as expendable hold another. Politicians, economists and even some philosophers tend to see things in purely utilitarian terms. Such people are likely to err on the side of treatment withdrawal and death. All these are vitally important and live issues in medical ethics.

Traditional palliative care

Palliative care came into being officially in the United Kingdom in 1987 when it received specialty status. The principles adopted by early practitioners can be found in a wide ranging article on symptom control by Robert Twycross, that was published in the British Journal of Hospital Medicine in 1986.[15] Dr Robert Twycross of Oxford, is well known for his opposition to euthanasia. His article showed the state of the art in those days, and was full of wisdom and practical advice for hospital doctors. The therapeutic and technical possibilities have increased in the intervening years but the principles remain the same. An extract from the article follows.

> Robert Twycross wrote- '*Symptom relief in patients who are close to death is an important and challenging part of most doctors' lives. It is difficult sometimes to accept that the battle for life has effectively been lost, and that life-sustaining measures are becoming progressively more futile and burdensome.*

5

'Most patients with a chronic, progressive, ultimately fatal disease have a clearly defined terminal phase. In relation to cancer it is the stage after anti-cancer treatment has been stopped. The emphasis in care has to shift from both prolongation of life and comfort to just comfort. There is commonly a period of transition rather than an abrupt change of direction in management. In the broad sense of the word such terminally ill patients are dying, but many do so slowly over weeks and months. Comments in this article have been restricted almost entirely to the malignant diseases.

Appropriate treatment. It should never be a matter of "to treat or not to treat?" but rather of what is the most appropriate treatment given the patient's biological prospects and personal and social circumstances. Appropriate treatment for an acutely ill patient is often inappropriate in the dying. Nasogastric tubes, intravenous infusions, antibiotics, cardiac resuscitation and artificial respiration are all primarily supportive measures for use in acute or acute-on-chronic illnesses to assist a patient through the initial period towards recovery of health. To use such measures in patients who are close to death and in whom there is no expectation of a return to health is usually inappropriate.[16]

'In deciding what is appropriate the following points should be borne in mind:
1. The patient's biological prospects
2. The therapeutic aim of the treatment
3. The need not to prescribe a lingering death.

Although the possibility of unexpected improvement or recovery should not be ignored, there are many occasions when it is appropriate to "give death a chance". All patients must die eventually: ultimately nature will take its course. In this respect the art of medicine is to decide when life sustenance is essentially futile and, therefore, when to allow death to occur without further impediment...' [15]

(Twycross © British Journal of Hospital Medicine 1986. Used with permission).

Terminally ill people as defined by the National Council for Hospice and Specialist Palliative Care Services (NCHSPCS) and the National Health Service Executive in 1995 are "those with active and progressive disease for which curative treatment is not possible or not appropriate, and from which death can reasonably be expected within twelve months." [17]

Palliative care

- Affirms life and regards dying as a normal process;
- Neither hastens nor postpones death:
- Provides relief from pain and other distressing symptoms:
- Integrates the psychological and spiritual aspects of patient care:
- Offers a support system to help patients live as actively as possible until death;
- Offers a support system to help the family cope during the patient's illness and in their own bereavement.[18,19.]

Palliative care as defined by the World Health Organisation (WHO) in 1990 is –
'The active and total care of patients whose disease is not responsive to curative treatment. Control of pain and other symptoms, and of psychological, social and spiritual problems is paramount. The goal of palliative care is achievement of the best quality of life for patients and their families. Many aspects of palliative care are also applicable in the earlier course of illness, in conjunction with anticancer treatment.'[18,19]

The WHO definition of palliative care as stated above, was quoted by the National Council for Hospice and Specialist Palliative Care Services (NCHSPCS) in their evidence to the House of Lords' Select Committee on Medical Ethics in 1993,[18] and was restated by others in 1997.[19] It paints an idealised, altruistic picture of the hospice movement as envisaged by Dame Cicely Saunders, revered pioneer of the hospice movement. For many patients and their relatives traditional palliative care is indeed a source of great comfort, but once in a while the experience is not a happy one.

Terminal sedation

Powerful sedative agents such as midazolam and methotrimeprazine are sometimes given by subcutaneous infusion to induce sedation in the terminal phase of life. They are used in patients who are distressed for one reason or another. The problem may be pain, or a terminal confusional state. No one can survive indefinitely without fluids or nourishment. Ethical problems arise if sedation is prolonged, and no artificial hydration is given, for the patient will eventually become dehydrated. A regime of sedation without hydration, dubbed "terminal sedation" or "slow euthanasia", raises important issues of morality, medicine and law that are explored in this book. The dividing line between killing and letting die can become gossamer thin. Rigid application of a policy of "comfort care only" in the dying is very dangerous.

Physicians in the United States of America may get a sense of 'déjà vue' on reading this book, for the ethical provision of nutrition and hydration in the dying has been a source of controversy and debate in North America for many years.[20-23] Despite almost two decades of debate, the subject remains highly charged and emotive simply because - as Siegler noted in 1987 - '*For physicians, provision of ordinary means of comfort and care - like food and water - demonstrates our personal, professional, and social commitment to the dying patient.*'[24]

The chapters that follow trace the course of the global debate, as launched afresh in the Journal of Medical Ethics in 1994

References

1. McNamara *et al.* Quoted by Corner J and Dunlop R. Ch. 18. New approaches to care. In New Themes in Palliative Care. Ed. Clark D, Hockley J, and Ahmedzai S. *Open University Press* 1997.
2. Auden W H. First things first. p.281. Collected shorter poems. *Faber and Faber*, London, 1966.

3. Fainsinger R, Bruera E. Hypodermoclysis (HDC) for Symptom control vs. the Edmonton Injector (EI). *Journal of Palliative Care.* 1991; **7**: 5-8.
4. Fainsinger R L, MacEarchern T, Miller M J. *et al.* The use of hypodermoclysis for rehydration in terminally ill cancer patients. *Journal of pain and symptom management.* 1994; **9**: 298-302.
5. Hoefler J M. Managing death. p.163. *Westgate Press.* 1997.
6. Gillon R. Euthanasia, withholding life-prolonging treatment, and moral difference between killing and letting die. (Editorial). *Journal of Medical Ethics.* 1988; **14**: 115-117.
7. Brown D. Choices. Chapter on euthanasia. p.125-131. *Blackwell.* 1983.
8. Craig G M. On withholding nutrition and hydration in the terminally ill. Has palliative medicine gone too far? *Journal of Medical Ethics.* 1994; **20**: 139-141.
9. Truog R D, Berde C B, Mitchell C. et al. Barbiturates in the care of the terminally ill. *New England Journal of Medicine.* 1992; **327**: 167-1682.
10. Janssens R J P A, Have H, Zylicz Z. Hospice and euthanasia in the Netherlands; an ethical point of view. *Journal of Medical Ethics.* 1999; **25**: 408-412.
11. Ramsay P. The Patient as a Person: Explorations in Medical Ethics. New Haven: *Yale University Press.* 1970.
12. Curran Charles E. On (only) caring for the dying, pages 152-163 in Politics, Medicine and Christian Ethics. *Fortress Press, Philadelphia* 1973.
13. Barth, K. quoted by Curran. Ref. 12 above, p.153.
14. Kelly G. quoted by Curran. Ibid. p.154.
15. Twycross R. Symptom control. *British Journal of Hospital Medicine* 1986, **36**: 244-249
16. Thompson I, In Palliative Care: The management of Far-Advanced Illness . Ed Doyle D. *Croom Helm, London*, 1986 p 461. Quoted by Twycross.
17. Guidelines on cardiopulmonary resuscitation. Note (1) *National Council for Hospice and Specialist Palliative Care Services,* July/August 1997.
18. Key ethical issues in palliative care. Evidence to House of Lords' Select Committee on Medical Ethics. Occasional Paper 3. *National Council for Hospice and Specialist Palliative Care Services. London.* July 1993.
19. O'Neill B, Fallon M. Principles of palliative care and pain control. *British Medical Journal* 1997; **315**: 801-804.
20. Thomasma D, Micetich K, Steinecker P. Continuance of nutritional care in the terminally ill patient. *Critical Care Clinics,* 1986; **2(1)**: 61-71.
21. Derr P. Why food and fluids can never be denied. *Hastings Centre Report* 1986; **16(1)**: 28-30.
22. Paris J. When burdens of feeding outweigh benefits. *Hastings Centre Report* 1986; **16(1)**: 30-32.
23. Billings J. Comfort measures for the terminally ill: is dehydration painful? *Journal of the American Geriatrics Society 1985*; **33(11)**: 808-810.
24. Siegler M, Schiedermayer D. Should fluid and nutritional support be withheld from terminally ill patients?- Tube feeding in hospice settings. *American Journal of Hospice Care*, 1987 March/April 32-35, at 35.

Chapter 2

The Debate in the Journal of Medical Ethics

Introduction.

The late Dr Jacob Bronowski once said "There is a time when we move from anonymous theoretical knowledge to personal open knowledge." That defining moment came for me during a week spent as an observer at the bedside of a man who was dying of cancer. I saw at first hand the practice of sedation without hydration and I was dismayed. Out of that experience grew a quiet determination to do what I could to change medical practice. Having surveyed the literature and discussed the issues in private with a number of senior members of the medical profession I was invited to write a paper for the Journal of Medical Ethics. I wrote the paper shortly before taking early retirement in 1993 and it was published in 1994 supported by a thoughtful editorial by Raanon Gillon, a commentary by Dr Eric Wilkes and a press release by the British Medical Association. The press release resulted in some interest in the media, with brief coverage in the Observer, The Daily Telegraph and on BBC Radio 5 Live. Thus the debate about the use of sedation without hydration in terminally ill patients was well and truly launched in the United Kingdom! The papers that launched the debate are reproduced in this chapter with the kind permission of the BMJ Publishing Group.

On withholding nutrition and hydration in the terminally ill: has palliative medicine gone too far?

Gillian M Craig. *Consultant Geriatrician, Northampton.*
Reprinted from Journal of Medical Ethics 1994 ; **20**:139-143.
© BMJ Publishing Group.

Author's abstract

This paper explores ethical issues relating to the management of patients who are terminally ill and unable to maintain their own nutrition and hydration. A policy of sedation without hydration or nutrition is used in palliative medicine under certain circumstances. The author argues that this policy is dangerous, medically, ethically and legally, and can be disturbing for relatives. The role of the family in management is discussed.

This issue requires wide debate by the public and the profession.

Introduction

From time to time in the professional life of a doctor incidents occur which cause one to stop and think. There are times when two doctors, each with the best interests of the patient at heart, would treat in diametrically opposite ways. There are widely divergent views about what is correct and morally acceptable when it comes to the management of patients who are, or appear to be, terminally ill and unable to maintain their own nutrition and hydration. This inability to eat and drink may be a consequence of the illness or of the treatment, for example heavy sedation. Differences in opinion about management may be voiced by relatives, by nurses and by doctors who may or may not be directly or professionally involved in the care of the patient. Particularly difficult management problems may arise if the dissenting relative is a nurse, doctor or paramedic, and great care must be taken to ensure that his or her views are taken into account and discussed openly, and that the management adopted is acceptable to all parties, if this is humanly and legally possible.

Ethical dilemmas in the field of hydration and nutrition cover a wide spectrum, from dehydration due to dysphagia of various aetiologies, through terminal cancer with intestinal obstruction, to the persistent vegetative state, terminal Alzheimer's disease patients who are unable to eat, and patients with anorexia nervosa or elderly depressives who deliberately refuse nourishment to the point of self-annihilation. The main issue highlighted by this paper is the use of sedation without hydration in the terminally ill. This raises ethical issues which require debate by the profession and the public.

The need for an open mind about intravenous hydration in terminal care

Palliative medicine is a relatively new and growing specialty and the hospice movement is held in high esteem by the public. Some doctors, however, have reservations. There are dangers in grouping patients labelled 'terminal' in institutions, because diagnoses can be wrong.[1] There is a risk that if all the staff in an institution are orientated towards death and dying and non-intervention, treatable illness may be overlooked. Not everyone who is referred for terminal care is terminally ill, and no physician should accept such a diagnosis without reviewing the evidence personally.

Certain policies that are practised in palliative medicine would be dangerous if applied without due care and thought. In particular the view that in the terminal phase of disease 'no form of artificial hydration or alimentation is undertaken, all measures not required for comfort are withdrawn, and no treatment-related toxicity is acceptable'[2]. It is not uncommon for the elderly to be admitted to hospital in a seriously dehydrated condition, looking terminally ill. A treatment-orientated physician will rehydrate these patients energetically, often with dramatic results, in order to buy time in which to assess the situation carefully. A therapeutically inactive doctor would lose many patients for the sake of avoiding a drip. Two examples from my personal experience will illustrate this point.

Case 1 An elderly man was sent to hospital for terminal care with a diagnosis of carcinoma of the pancreas. He had indeed had a stent inserted at another hospital to relieve biliary obstruction due to tumour. However his 'terminal' illness was due to a small stroke and uncontrolled diabetes mellitus. He recovered with insulin and intravenous rehydration and lived happily for several weeks more.

Case 2 An elderly man was admitted for terminal care but the geriatrician felt the diagnosis of cancer was not well established. The main problem was severe dehydration with ischaemic feet and severe pressure sores on the heels. With intravenous rehydration and intensive nursing he recovered and went home for eighteen months.

It is important for the public to realise that most patients with terminal illness can continue to eat and drink as and when they wish. Only in the last days may they be too weak or tired to bother, in which case the lack of food and drink will not contribute to death. If dehydration develops under these circumstances it is a natural consequence of irreversible disease, and artificial hydration would not be appropriate.

The use of sedation.

There are times in the care of the dying 'when it is necessary to use benzodiazepines, phenothiazines and barbiturates to sedate a patient in order to relieve intolerable distress where dying is complicated by an agitated delirium or tracheal obstruction'.[3] In skilled hands no person should die in pain, whatever the cause of the illness. As a last resort some advocate the use of high-dose analgesia and induction of sleep with continuous intravenous midazolam.[4] Whatever the underlying pathology 'the cardinal ethical principle remains that the treatment goal must be achieved with the least risk to the patient's life'.[3] I would add - and in a manner that is acceptable to the patient's closest relatives.

Having decided that sedation is needed, the doctor must try to find a drug regime that relieves distress but does not prevent the patient from taking fluid and nourishment, does not prevent verbal communication with friends and relatives, and does not lead to toxic side- effects or expedite death. Unfortunately currently available therapeutic options are not ideal in all these respects. Even light sedation can cause drowsiness that may prevent a person from taking enough fluid to maintain hydration. Heavy sedation may render an alert person incapable of swallowing within minutes, depending on the drug regime used.

If death is imminent few people would feel it essential to put up a drip but ethical problems arise if sedation is continued for more than one or two days, without hydration, as the patient will become dehydrated. Dehydration can result in circulatory collapse, renal failure, anuria and death. I do not think that it is morally acceptable to leave a sedated patient for long without hydration. Others would dissent from this view using words such as 'meddlesome' and 'unethical' if intravenous fluids are suggested under such circumstances. However, in my opinion, if it is not possible to reduce sedation to a level that enables the patient to drink, the question of hydration must be addressed to everyone's satisfaction.

Particular problems may arise if the patient has a primary mental disorder such as chronic schizophrenia or depression. In such people the stress of the physical illness may make the mental state worse. Great skill may be needed to distinguish a potentially treatable psychotic reaction from an untreatable, terminal agitated delirium. In cases of difficulty expert psychiatric help should be obtained as the distinction may be vital. If the diagnosis is a psychotic reaction, hydration must be maintained and the patient observed in the hope that sedation can be reduced. If the diagnosis is a terminal agitated delirium, those with experience advise against reducing sedation, and argue against giving intravenous fluids as this would prolong dying.

To take a decision to sedate a person, without hydration, until he/she dies is a very dangerous policy medically, ethically and legally. No doctor's judgement is infallible when it comes to predicting how close a person is to death. To say that it is a matter of days, and to treat by this method, is to make the prophecy self-fulfilling. I know of a patient who died after at least seven days of sedation without hydration - how much longer would he have lived with hydration? Diagnostic errors can also occur. A reversible psychosis or confusional state can be mistaken for terminal delirium, aspiration pneumonia for tracheal obstruction, obstruction due to faecal impaction for something more sinister, and so on. The only way to ensure that life will not be shortened is to maintain hydration in all cases where inability to eat and drink is a direct consequence of sedation, unless the relatives request no further intervention, or the patient has made his or her wishes known to this effect. If naturally or artificially administered hydration and nutrition is withheld, the responsible medical staff must face the fact that prolonged sedation without hydration or nutrition will end in death, whatever the underlying pathology. Even a fit Bedu tribesman riding in the desert in cool weather, can only survive for seven days without food or water.[5]

The legal question

The Institute of Medical Ethics working party on the ethics of prolonging life and assisting death has argued the case for withdrawing food and water from patients in a persistent vegetative state.[6] Such patients are unaware of their surroundings as a result of severe brain damage. Recent reports indicate that 'persistent' does not necessarily mean 'permanent' [7] and it is essential to ensure that the prognosis is hopeless before considering withdrawing treatment.[8]

A key issue in English law in such patients has been 'whether artificial feeding counts as medical treatment - which can lawfully be discontinued if the patient is receiving no benefit - or is simply the means of sustaining life, which if withdrawn could lay a doctor open to a charge of murder'.[8] This argument is largely semantic since in patients with a persistent vegetative state this treatment sustains life. The key issue surely is whether it benefits the patient to be alive rather than dead. Those who advocate withdrawing food and water from these patients have been warned by medical defence organisations that such a policy may result in a charge of manslaughter by neglect.[9] This risk has been reduced but not eliminated by the Bland case ruling [10] which has clarified the legal position in England and Wales. The legal position in Scotland remains unclear but is being actively reviewed by the Lord Advocate following the judgement in the Bland case.*

The case of Airedale NHS Trust v Bland

In the final judgement or declaratory statement made in the House of Lords in February 1993, it was ruled that the responsible attending physicians could lawfully discontinue life-sustaining treatment and medical supportive measures designed to keep the patient (Mr Bland) alive in his persistent vegetative state, including the termination of ventilation, nutrition and hydration by artificial means.[10] In coming to this judgement, the Law Lords accepted as responsible medical opinion, a paper prepared by the British Medical Association (BMA) Medical Ethics Committee.[11] Referring to this the judges highlighted four safeguards which should be observed before discontinuing life support in a patient with a persistent vegetative state- namely, 1. Every effort should be made to rehabilitate for at least six months after injury; 2. The diagnosis of persistent vegetative state should not be considered confirmed until at least 12 months after injury; 3. The diagnosis should be agreed by at least two other independent doctors, and 4. Generally the wishes of the patient's immediate family should be given great weight.

Lord Goff pointed out that to discontinue artificial feeding might be categorised as an omission, which if deemed to constitute a breach of duty to the patient is unlawful.[10] However, in the case of Mr Bland, he argued that the patient was incapable of swallowing and therefore of eating and drinking in the normal sense of these words. Artificial feeding via a naso-gastric tube was therefore a form of life support, and could be discontinued if treatment was futile and no longer in the best interests of the patient.

It must be emphasised that the case of Airedale NHS Trust v Bland does not give doctors freedom to withdraw treatment from all patients in a persistent vegetative state. For the foreseeable future doctors in England and Wales must apply to the family division of the High Court for a declaration in each case as to the legality of any proposed discontinuance of life support, where there is no valid consent on the part of the patient. There has not been a rush of applications to date. Moreover a civil court ruling is no guarantee against subsequent prosecution in a criminal court, since a declaration as to the lawfulness or otherwise of future conduct is 'no bar to a criminal prosecution, no matter the authority of the court which grants it'.[12]

The judgement regarding hydration and nutrition in the Bland case was clearly swayed by the patient's irreversible brain damage, although the law as

* (For outcome see p.63 of this book).

to killing is unaffected by the victim's mental state.[13] It would be extremely dangerous to extrapolate the legal decision made in this case to other clinical situations. The legality or otherwise of withholding hydration and nutrition from the dying has not been tested in the Courts in the United Kingdom.[13]

Despite the differences in mental state, pathology and life expectancy between a terminally ill sedated patient and one with a persistent vegetative state, the key issues are similar. Are you, by withholding fluid and nourishment, withholding the means of sustaining life? In short are you killing the patient? The answer I fear in some cases could be YES. In some terminally ill patients, especially those who are rendered unable to swallow by heavy sedation, failure to hydrate and nourish artificially could be judged an unlawful omission. The question of intent is important and the principle of double effect, and other medico-legal issues are relevant.[13] However doctors who deliberately speed death could face the prospect of life imprisonment.[13] Clearly the legality of prolonged sedation without hydration is highly debatable yet this treatment is regarded as ethical and compassionate by senior and respected specialists in palliative medicine. If a dying patient is treated in this way there may be reasonable grounds for doubt as to whether the patient died of the treatment or the disease. It is our duty and our privilege as doctors to sustain life, not to shorten it. Euthanasia must remain illegal, and practices that seem tantamount to euthanasia must be exposed.

The risk of inappropriate sedation

Clearly a policy of sedation without hydration or nutrition in palliative care is a drastic solution to a difficult problem. Those who take such action no doubt do so thinking that they have the patient's best interests at heart. They may also be influenced by subconscious fears. As Main said: 'Perhaps many of the desperate treatments in medicine can be justified by expediency, but history has an awkward habit of judging some as fashions, more helpful to the therapist than the patient. Patients tend to be sedated when the carers have reached the end of their resources, and are no longer able to stand the patient's problems without anxiety, impatience, guilt, anger or despair. A sedative will alter the situation and produce a patient who if not dead, is al least quiet'.[14] The case of the Winchester rheumatologist who was convicted of attempted murder demonstrates what can happen when doctor and patient reach the end of their tether.[15,19]

The importance of comfort

The guiding principle in the care of the dying is that 'everything in the terminal phase of an irreversible illness should be clearly decided on the basis of whether it will make the patient more comfortable and whether it will honour his/her wishes'.[17] 'Comfort' is a state of conscious physical and mental well-being. It is debatable therefore whether the word can be applied to a heavily sedated, dehydrated patient. However, most would agree that it is preferable to be comfortable and conscious or semi-conscious without pain, than uncomfortable, distraught and fully awake.

The therapeutic ideal would be to have a patient who is calm, clear-headed and pain-free. Unfortunately there are times when this cannot be achieved with the drugs at our disposal.

The consensus in the hospice movement seems to be that rehydration and intravenous fluids are inappropriate in terminal care [2,18,19]. Dehydration is even considered to be beneficial in patients with incontinence! [18] This is a weak argument to justify withholding intravenous fluids. Therapeutic anuria may be the ultimate cure for incontinence but the side-effect is death. Those who have coped with incontinence without a catheter in the past can be nursed without a catheter to the end, if that is their wish. Rehydration should not influence this aspect of care. Hospice staff also argue that a drip makes it difficult to turn a dying patient, yet they are happy to give analgesics by subcutaneous infusion when necessary, and occasionally use a drip in patients with hypercalcaemia. To those who use drips frequently on acute medical, surgical and geriatric wards, these arguments do not carry much weight. Setting up a drip or a subcutaneous infusion is a simple and straightforward procedure that rarely causes the patient discomfort or distress. Many dehydrated patients look and feel a lot better when they are rehydrated. If the staff in hospices used drips more, they would not have to find so many reasons for avoiding them.

The question of thirst

If hydration and nutrition are withheld, the attendant staff must be sensitive to the effect this may have on the family and friends.[17] Some say that a patient should be comatose, so as not to experience thirst, before it is morally acceptable to withhold or withdraw intravenous fluids.[20] It is widely assumed that a terminally ill patient is not troubled by hunger or thirst but this is difficult to substantiate as few people return from the grave to complain. Thirst may or may not bother the patient. Concern about thirst undoubtedly bothers relatives. They will long to give their loved one a drink. They may sit by the bed furtively drinking cups of tea, taking care to make no sound lest the clink of china is torture to the patient. Anyone who has starved for hours before an anaesthetic will sympathise with dying patients who seem to thirst and starve for days. Nurses are taught that moistening the patient's mouth with a damp sponge is all that is necessary to prevent thirst. Relatives may not be convinced. It may well be that sedation relieves the sensation of hunger or thirst. If there is evidence to this effect it would be helpful for the relatives of dying patients to be told about it.

The role of the family

It has been said that the family must request no further medical procedures before treatment can be withheld and that the previously expressed wishes of the patient or current family must predominate over those of staff.[20] Staff who believe strongly that intravenous fluids are inappropriate should not impose their views on knowledgeable or distressed relatives who request that a dying patient be given intravenous fluids to prevent dehydration or thirst. To overrule such a request is, in my view, ethically wrong. The only proviso would be if the patient had, when *compos mentis*, specifically said that he/she did not want a drip under any circumstances.

No relatives should be forced to watch a loved one die while medical staff insist on withholding hydration. This has happened to my knowledge. Such an experience is deeply disturbing and could haunt a person forever. Is all this agony worth it for the sake of avoiding a drip? I think not.

The converse also applies. There will be occasions when the medical staff who are professionally involved would like to use a drip, but a knowledgeable relative requests no intervention. In this situation, the medical team will make a carefully balanced judgement as to whether intervention is essential or not. If the scales are not heavily weighted in favour of intervention the wise doctor will compromise and stand back in the interests of the peace of mind of the relative.

A doctor cannot be obliged to act contrary to his or her own conscience but equally doctors should bear in mind that relatives also have consciences, and should not be forced to accept for their loved ones treatment that they consider to be unethical. It is inevitable that terminally ill patients will die and that their relatives will be sad. Care must be taken to ensure that the burden of bereavement is not loaded heavily by distress about patient management in the terminal phase. In the care of the dying, both patients and their relatives must be treated with compassion.

Final comments

The question of hydration and nutrition in terminal care is one that generates strong views. It is probably inevitable that sooner or later those working in the field of palliative care will meet colleagues working in different fields of medicine who are used to adopting a more active approach to management. Those who don't believe in using intravenous fluids will encounter those who do. Faced with this situation it is essential that both parties sit down together to discuss the issues. They must reach a compromise that takes into account the expressed or probable wishes of the patient concerned and the views of the closest relatives. No one individual has right entirely on his/her side. The ethically correct solution may prove to be somewhere in the middle, and it must be found.

Where opinions differ on the management of an individual case, further discussion may throw light on the situation, firmly held opinions may prove to be wrong, diagnoses may need to be revised and factors that had not been considered before may soften entrenched attitudes. If the issue is the futility or otherwise of intervention, or doubt about the patient's views or best interest, there may be room for manoeuvre in any given situation. The underlying reasons for sedation and the cause of the patient's inability to eat and drink are obviously of critical importance. What is essential in the final analysis is that all parties should feel comfortable with the clinical management strategy adopted. If this is not the case the strategy is probably not ethically sound. Somewhere between the poles of opposing opinion there must be some morally acceptable common ground. If after further discussion a mutually acceptable management policy cannot be agreed, it is no solution to the dilemma for a hospice team to tell the relatives to take the patient elsewhere. Where for example can you take a dying man, in the middle of winter, in an ambulance strike? However strong your ethical position, it is unacceptable to seek to silence dissent in this way. Where time permits, a second consultant opinion should be sought, or help from some appropriate independent source.

As Rabbi Lionel Blue said recently of theology: 'Even more important than your own views is the kindness with which you hold them, and the courtesy with which you treat those who oppose you'. The same could be said of the issues explored in this paper. People who hold strong views in this difficult and emotive area of palliative medicine should hold them kindly and with sensitivity. At the end of the day there should not be the slightest grounds for suspicion that death was due to anything but the disease. Unless this can be guaranteed, the public's faith in doctors in general, and in the hospice movement in particular, will be ill founded.

Gillian Craig, MD, FRCP, is a retired Consultant Geriatrician.

References

1. Kamisar Y. In Downing A. ed. *Euthanasia and the right to death.* London: Peter Owen, 1969:100-101.
2. Ashby M, Stoffell B. Therapeutic ratio and defined phases: proposal of ethical framework for palliative care. *British medical journal* 1991;302:1322-1324.
3. Twycross R G Assisted death: a reply. *Lancet* 1990; 336:796-798.
4. Tapsfield W, Amis P (letter). *British medical journal* 1992; 305: 951.
5. Thesiger W. *Arabian sands.* London: Readers' Union, Longmans, Green and Co, 1960:87.
6. Institute of Medical Ethics working party on the ethics of prolonging life and assisting death. Withdrawal of life support from patients in a persistent vegetative state. *Lancet* 1991; 337: 96-98.
7. Andrews K. Managing the persistent vegetative state. *British medical journal* 1992; 305: 486-487.
8. Dyer C. BMA examines the persistent vegetative state. *British medical journal* 1992; 305: 853-854.
9. Baron J H (letter). *Lancet* 1991; 337: 639.
10. House of Lords. Law Report. Withdrawal of medical treatment from hopeless case not unlawful. *The Times* 1993 Feb 5:8.
11. Medical Ethics Committee of the British Medical Association. Discussion paper on treatment of patients in a persistent vegetative state. London: *BMA,* 1992.

12. See reference 10: Viscount Dilhorne in Imperial Tobacco Ltd. v Attorney General 1981.AC. 718 741 Quoted by Lord Goff.
13. Mason J K, McCall Smith R A. *Law and medical ethics* (3rd ed.) London: *Butterworths,* 1991: 317-343.
14. Main T F. The ailment. *British journal of medical psychology* 1957; 30: 129-145.
15. Dyer C. Rheumatologist convicted of attempted murder. *British medical journal* 1992; 305: 731.
16. Illidge T M, Kirkham S R (letter). *British medical journal* 1992; 305: 1225.
17. Wanzer S H, Adelstein S J, Cranford R E. *et al.* The physician's responsibility towards hopelessly ill patients. *New England Journal of Medicine* 1984; 310: 955-959.
18. Sykes N. The last 48 hours of life: caring for patient, family and doctor. *Geriatric medicine* 1990; 20, 9: 22-24.
19. Belcher N G. Pulling out the drip: an ethical decision in the terminally ill. *Geriatric medicine* 1990; 20, 6: 22-23.
20. Micetich K C, Steinecker P H, Thomasma D C *et al.* Are intravenous fluids morally required for a dying patient? *Archives of internal medicine* 1983; 143: 975-978.

Dr. Craig's paper was supported by a thoughtful and wide-ranging editorial by Raanon Gillon, a highly respected British medical ethicist, who was at the time editor of the Journal of Medical Ethics. Eric Wilkes, then Consultant Adviser to Trent Region Palliative and Continuing Care Centre provided a commentary. The text of their papers as published in the Journal of Medical Ethics in 1994 is reprinted below with the kind permission of the BMJ Publishing Group.

Editorial Palliative care ethics: non-provision of artificial nutrition and hydration to terminally ill sedated patients

Raanon Gillon. Imperial College Health Service and St. Mary's College Hospital Medical School, London University.
Reprinted from Journal of Medical Ethics 1994; **20**; 131-132.
© BMJ Publishing Group.

In this issue of the journal Dr Gillian Craig [1] and her commentator Dr Eric Wilkes [2] raise a variety of important questions about ethical aspects of palliative care medicine that deserve careful reflection. Perhaps the most difficult and contentious of the issues raised by Dr Craig are (a) the question of withholding or withdrawing of artificial nutrition and hydration from terminally ill patients who, because of pain or severe suffering, have been sedated; and (b) the question of how to deal with disagreement between the patient's health care workers and the patient's family members, if this arises when the patient cannot be consulted directly.

So far as the first question is concerned, Dr Craig is clear that except at the time of actual dying (easier to identify in retrospect than in prospect), 'I do not think that it is morally acceptable to leave a sedated patient for long without hydration'- by which, the context makes clear, she means that if the patient is too sedated to take sufficient fluids by mouth then a drip should be put up so as to attain the normal medical standards of adequate hydration. As she also writes, 'Others would dissent from this view using words such as "meddlesome" and "unethical" if intravenous fluids are suggested under such circumstances'. However, so far as she is concerned, 'To take a decision to sedate a person, without hydration, until he/she dies is a very dangerous policy, medically, ethically and legally'.

For Dr Craig 'The only way to ensure that a life will not be shortened is to maintain hydration during sedation in all cases where inability to eat and drink is a direct consequence of sedation, unless the relatives request no further intervention, or if the patient has made his/her wishes known to this effect... the responsible medical staff must face the fact that prolonged sedation without hydration or nutrition will end in death, whatever the underlying pathology' and she points out that 'even a fit Bedu tribesman riding in the desert in cool weather can only survive for seven days without food or water'.

The issues of killing and letting die have been addressed before in these columns.[3-4] In summary, while it has been very thoroughly demonstrated by example and philosophical argument that there is no necessary moral distinction to be drawn between killing and letting die, they are not necessarily morally equivalent. Moral distinctions between killing and letting die may arise:

- As a result of religious commitments;
- As a result of legal obligations
- As a result of differences in the overall benefits and harms resulting from policies that forbid all intentional killings (of non-aggressors) versus those that would result from policies that would also forbid all intentional allowings to die.
- As a result of differences in the motives and intentions of the agent, and
- As a result of differences in the duties of care owed by the agents to the persons who are killed or allowed to die.

In practical ethical terms, doctors are both morally and legally justified in withholding or withdrawing treatments that are not beneficial to their patients, and are morally and legally required to withhold or withdraw any treatments that are harmful.

The fact that withholding or withdrawing non-beneficial or positively harmful medical interventions would, or might, result in the patient's death earlier than would otherwise have been the case if the medical intervention had been instituted or maintained does not, it is widely agreed, demonstrate that such withholding or withdrawing is either wrong or illegal.[5-10] On the contrary, as the lawyer Professor Skegg put it, 'Doctors are sometimes free- sometimes indeed required- to allow a patient to die'.[11] Thus, *pace* Dr Craig, concern about 'the only way to ensure that a life will not be shortened' is widely held to be less important than the traditional medico-moral objective of benefiting the patient with minimal harm; and the legal translation of this into the doctor's obligation to fulfil his or her duty of care. Artificial hydration and nutrition may or may not be ways of fulfilling those moral and legal obligations.

While in normal circumstances it is in principle possible to ask the patient about his or her preferences concerning such treatment- and different patients in similar predicaments may well have very different preferences- Dr Craig raises four important complicating concerns. The first is the terminally ill patient who is sedated because of severe distress and/or pain. The second is the terminally ill patient who is also mentally ill and who is sedated because of increased agitation caused either by deterioration in the primary mental disorder or by the agony of impending death- so called terminal agitated delirium. The third complicating factor is disagreement about the appropriate management between, on the one hand the medical and nursing staff, and on the other hand close members of the patient's family. And Dr Craig's fourth complicating factor concerns family members who disagree with the medical carers who are themselves medically qualified or otherwise medically 'knowledgeable'.

A variety of guidelines are available to help medical and nursing staff in such cases, whether in hospices or hospitals.[6-9] The Appleton international consensus guidelines,[8] similar to the British Medical Association (BMA) guidelines, make it clear that the patient's own views are preferable where available and willingly provided. Where the patient is not sufficiently mentally competent for such discussion to be reliable, it may be possible to reduce the sedation or otherwise wait for a lucid period in which the patient's autonomous views may be obtained. If not, relatives or friends may function as proxy. Where this has not happened, those close to the patient, preferably those who are in a position to know what the patient's own values and preferences would be, should be consulted.

As the BMA advise,[6] in deciding whether life-prolonging treatment is in the best interests of the patient the health team should consider three main factors:

- The possibility of extending life under humane and comfortable conditions.
- The patient's values about life and the way it should be lived, and
- The patient's likely reaction to sickness, suffering and medical intervention.

And the BMA add that 'although doctors should not give treatment simply because it is available, in cases of doubt about the best interests of the patient, the presumption should be in favour of prolonging life. This is particularly so if most people would consider that life to be of acceptable quality'.[6]

Thus, when the patient is unable (or unwilling) to provide information about his or her own preferences, doctors should try to consult a family member or close friend who knows the patient's own views.

In cases of disagreement between doctors and patients' proxies, whether family or friends, the BMA recommend 'counselling, discussion and further medical opinion', with time and effort being put into resolving the conflict, and a preference for avoiding the need to go to court.[6] The Appleton and the Hastings guidelines add that some form of conflict-resolving mechanism should be in place. Like the BMA, the Appleton consensus recommends in the first instance 'counselling, discussion, consultation and other informal interventions'. If there is disagreement between different members of the patient's family or circle of friends, then doctors should prefer the advice of those who are 'emotionally and socially close' to the patient and 'may disregard the claims of the more tangential party'. If, however, disagreement remains with someone close to the patient then 'the physician should not generally override that view without resorting to more formal conflict resolution processes'.[8]

The sort of conflicts alluded to by Dr Craig seem precisely the sort that would require formal mediation. One can imagine a situation in which a medically qualified family member feels outraged by the proposed management of a severely disturbed terminally ill close relative by sedation and the withholding of artificial nutrition and hydration. One can equally well imagine the response of the medical team to a proposal by a medically qualified family member that the patient ought to have a drip. As suggested by Dr Wilkes in his commentary, 'we need to be tactfully resistant to sacrificing the interests of our patient to the emotional distress of the relatives'.[2]

However, should it come to a straightforward unresolvable disagreement between a relative acting as proxy and the health care team about whether prolonging the life of a terminally ill patient by artificial hydration is in the patient's interests, then it seems important for the dispute to be referred to some sort of formal mediation procedure. Is it not time that British hospitals and hospices developed such procedures? There certainly seems no obvious reason to assume that in such disputes the doctors and medical teams are always right, if indeed there is a clearly 'right' answer. But even if the doctors were always or usually right, not only should justice be done, it should also be seen to be done.

References

1. Craig G.. Withholding nutrition and hydration in the terminally ill: has palliative medicine gone too far? *Journal of medical ethics* 1994; 20: 139-143.
2. Wilkes E. On withholding nutrition and hydration in the terminally ill: has palliative medicine gone too far? A commentary. *Journal of medical ethics* 1994; 20: 144-145.
3. Anon: (editorial). Acts and omissions: killing and letting die. *Journal of medical ethics* 1984; 2: 59-60.

4. Gillon R. Euthanasia, withholding life-prolonging treatment, and moral differences between killing and letting die. *Journal of medical ethics* 1988; 14: 115-117.
5. Kennedy I, Grubb A eds. *Medical Law: texts and materials.* London: Butterworths, 1989: 1074, and more generally, 1066-1055.
6. British Medical Association. *Medical ethics today- its practice and philosophy.* London: BMJ publishing group, 1993: 165, and more generally, 147-179.
7. President's Commission for the study of ethical problems in medicine and biomedical and behavioural research. *Deciding to forego life-sustaining treatment- ethical, medical and legal issues in treatment decisions.* Washington, DC: US Government Printing Office, 1983: 90, and more generally, 43-90.
8. Stanley J, ed. The Appleton international conference: developing guidelines for decisions to forego life-prolonging medical treatment. *Journal of medical ethics* (supp) 1992; 18: 1-24.
9. Hastings Centre. *Guidelines on the termination of life-sustaining treatment and the care of the dying.* Briarcliff Manor, NY: The Hasting Centre, 1987: 60, 16-34.
10. Lynn J. Introduction and overview. In Lynn J, ed. *By no extraordinary means - the choice to forgo life-sustaining food and water.* Bloomington, Indianapolis: Indiana University Press, 1986: 4.
11. Skegg P. *Law, ethics and medicine–studies in medical law.* Oxford: Clarendon Press, 1984:143.

Despite the passage of time, the points made by Raanon Gillon in 1994 remain valid. Sedation without hydration is still practiced at the end of life under some circumstances. Decisions to withhold life-prolonging fluids and nutrition given by artificial means such as tube feeding are increasingly common especially in elderly stroke patients who have lost the ability to swallow. Conflict resolution procedures within the National Health Service remain rudimentary and unsatisfactory. Proxy decision makers have legal standing in the United States of America, but not in the United Kingdom at present- but this may change if the Mental Capacity Bill published in June 2004 becomes law.

The British Medical Association guidelines of 1993, to which Professor Gillon referred, have been overtaken by their guidelines of 1999 on 'Withholding and Withdrawing Life-Prolonging Medical Treatment' and by similar General Medical Council guidelines of August 2002. The National Council for Hospice and Specialist Palliative Care Services published guidelines on the ethical use of artificial hydration in the terminally ill in 1997 and the American Medical Association issued guidance on conflict resolution in March 1999. All these guidelines and related issues will be discussed later in this book or in Volume 2.

On withholding nutrition and hydration in the terminally ill: has palliative medicine gone too far? A commentary.

Eric Wilkes

Consultant Advisor to Trent Region Palliative and Continuing Care Centre.
Reprinted from the Journal of Medical Ethics 1994; 20: 144-145.
© BMJ Publishing Group.

One has to share some of Dr Craig's anxieties. We must strive for an accurate diagnosis for those who have not long to live or we cannot provide all possible help for them. But we know that hospice physicians create more routine investigations and a balance between over-investigation and neglect in the care of the dying is not easily achieved. I remember Dame Albertine Winner saying that a cup of tea is of much more use than a blood count in such cases.

Accurate diagnosis in hospice patients is usually straightforward. Admission should be preceded by careful clinical assessment and a full medical report. A hospice is no place for solving diagnostic problems, but so long as over ninety-five percent of admissions are to do with disseminated and inoperable malignant disease, this presents few difficulties.

Even so, during my 15 years as a medical director of a busy hospice occasionally humiliating lessons had to be learned; but these were more often cases of unexpected survival- the breast cancer patient whose skeletal abnormalities turned out to be due to Paget's Disease, for example- rather than errors associated with mismanagement and a premature death. I remember only one case of leukaemia, many years ago, that seemed to have inadequate therapy. Our referral to a different specialist unit led to further treatment and the pleasure of seeing the patient's case demonstrated at a grand round several years later as 'a cure referred by the hospice'. That must be very rare.

Indeed hospice colleagues tell me that they still see more of enthusiastic over-treatment than of neglect. There are implications here for hospital training that sooner or later will need to be addressed and for hospice training too, as palliative care moves towards mainstream medicine. The fact that old age is the time for multiple pathologies as well as for dying means that the training of the hospice physician must have a generalist approach. If we take even half seriously the aspirations of the recent Standing Medical Advisory Committee and Standing Nursing and Midwifery Advisory Committee paper, *Principles and Provision of Palliative Care,*[1] the expertise in the symptom control of advanced cancer will not be enough. Some geriatric and rehabilitation skills will also be required, the management of advanced AIDS and Motor Neurone Disease, of secondary diagnoses such as renal failure or uncontrolled diabetes, all must be part of our stock in trade.

Palliative care is essentially a multi-disciplinary effort, and although the diffusion of hospice responsibilities will occur only slowly and with difficulty, analogous problems await our nursing colleagues for which they are not yet prepared.

If their patient has only a short time to live the problem of excessive dependence is irrelevant: but a disabled sufferer from, say, multiple sclerosis must be helped to cope with years of survival and patients encouraged to dress themselves even if it is exhausting and takes a long time. That would be cruel and unacceptable for the breathless lung cancer patient. It is difficult to combine these two different cultural attitudes on the same ward.

There are two tendencies to be observed in the present background to palliative care. First, the crudities of the 'contract culture' may threaten the survival of costly hospice units. Second, if staffing levels are lowered and our responsibilities widened to take in the whole spectrum of incurable illness, the new specialty of palliative medicine will have its expertise dangerously diluted.

It may well be therefore that Dr Craig's points are not to be taken too seriously- yet: but they point the way to problems that will be with us for a long time and will not be easily resolved.

Dying is a social act. Usually even in the presence of grief, there should be little in the way of anger or resentment directed at the carers by those about to be bereaved so long as they are informed and involved as fully as possible in the management of the case. The health professionals need to be aware that every casual phrase, any inevitable difficulties, the minutest details, are likely to be recalled by the family to the end of their days- influencing attitudes and giving comfort or distress for many years. This makes information and effective communication essential. Generally the process is both easy and rewarding.

But there are always exceptions and we need to be tactfully resistant to sacrificing the interests of our patients to the emotional distress of the relatives. An old man, transferred to a hospice after a hospital transfusion, was gently going downhill, but this caused sufficient distress to the son for him to demand: 'Can't you do more for my father? He's only ninety-two'.

Such poor adjustment to dying can be found in all walks of life, although those who have a tough life in the city or on the farm quite often cope better than the doctor or the priest when they have to face the death of someone close. But everyone can feel excluded and ignored if all the measures that might prolong the process of dying are not deployed.

Sometimes patients come to a hospice seeking sanctuary from modern medicine, such as respite from their chemotherapy. Others may be desperate to continue their chemotherapy for all that in their case it may be little more than a toxic or costly placebo. All doctors will therefore have to walk the tight-rope between over-treatment and neglect. The comfort of the patient must come first. Two common threats to the comfort of the dying are chest infections and dehydration, so perhaps they merit special mention.

Pneumonia was called, significantly enough in the last century, the old man's friend, for so often it put an end to suffering. Today in modern palliative care the chest infection in the incurably ill may be an intercurrent infection causing fever, cough, breathlessness so as to merit treatment under the heading of symptom-control. Alternatively it can be the beginning of the process of dying and not therefore to be officiously prolonged. Usually the difference is readily obvious, especially if colleagues and carers are involved in the assessment. The previously expressed opinions and wishes of the patient can be both helpful and relevant.

But rarely there will be doubt and here a delay of a day in the initiation of antibiotic treatment can either make the desirability of energetic treatment clear or it can see the patient moving speedily towards death. Where there is still doubt, the patient should have the benefit of it.

Near the beginning of my career as a hospice physician, when the patient's symptoms were well controlled and they were resting peacefully, as they moved nearer to death I would tend to reduce the dosage. This too often was associated with a restlessness as patients surfaced close to a reality with which they could no longer cope. The regime necessary to control distress was therefore maintained to the end. A comatose patient was much the lesser evil, yet despite encouraging nurses and carers to give small sips of water, dehydration could occur. Indeed, it sadly occurs far too frequently on medical and surgical wards far removed from the territory of palliative care.

In a hospice one is properly anxious to avoid either intravenous or subcutaneous infusions unless the needs are clear, for these can medicalise the process of dying, inhibit the limited mobility of the patient, and impede the involvement of the relatives. But in a sedated patient such infusions may be necessary to control discomfort or prevent infection. This is not often necessary and can be made even rarer by the overnight insertion of a slow drip of rectal tapwater when it has proved difficult to maintain oral intake of fluids. This homely remedy still has its place, especially as dehydration can distress the more aware relatives and sour their relationships with the carer to what may seem a disproportionate degree.

Eric Wilkes, OBE, FRCP, FRCGP, FRCPsych, was at the time of publication Consultant Adviser to Trent Region Palliative and Continuing Care Centre in the UK. He has now retired.

Reference

1. *The principles and provision of palliative care.* Joint report of the Standing Medical Advisory Committee and Standing Nursing and Midwifery Advisory Committee. London: HMSO, 1992.

Chapter 3

The Role of Hydration in the Care of the Dying: An Overview of the Debate

Author Gillian Craig.

Introduction

This chapter traces the progress of the debate between 1994 and 1998, and shows how palliative carers in the United Kingdom and beyond responded to criticism voiced in the Journal of Medical Ethics. The debate developed in several phases:-

1. Distribution of reprints by the author, with a covering letter to key individuals.
2. Informal discussion of the issues in hospices.
3. Publication of further papers, formal responses and correspondence in the Journal of Medical Ethics and other professional journals.
4. Publication of new textbooks on palliative care.
5. A hidden debate behind the scenes in committee rooms as guidelines were thrashed out.
6. Publication of guidelines on the ethical use of artificial hydration in terminally ill patients in 1997.
7. Debate at conferences organised by the Royal College of Physicians and other organisations in 1997 and 1998.

The hydration debate has raised many important questions that will be explored later in the book, for example-

- Should there be a more active approach to hydration in the dying?
- Is it legal, ethical and medically correct to sedate a dying patient who is mentally distressed, or in severe pain? The answer is clearly "Yes". If the patient is mentally unable to give consent to this treatment whose responsibility is it to do so?
- If sedation relieves the distress or pain but the patient is unable to drink, the patient will become dehydrated. Since untreated dehydration is fatal, can a refusal to give artificial hydration to a dehydrated patient amount to criminal negligence or murder?
- What does it feel like to be a patient dying of dehydration? Is there extreme thirst and discomfort? Palliative carers suggest that this may not be so, but the evidence does not appear to be strong.
- What does it feel like to be a relative, obliged to watch a loved one die under such circumstances? Some who realise what is happening are deeply distressed and may suffer post-traumatic stress.
- What happens when relatives complain? Do they get a fair hearing, or are they brushed aside? Examples will be given to illustrate what can happen.
- Is there a workable system for resolving disputes between dissenting relatives/ friends and health care decision makers during the life of the patient?

The answer to the last question in the U.K. is regrettably "No, not yet". The National Health Service complaints procedure is highly unsatisfactory. Those who seek redress through the courts face a lengthy, complex and expensive legal system, so many deserving cases never see the light of day.

The initial response

Following the publication of papers in the Journal of medical ethics in 1994.[1-3] I endeavoured to promote debate by distributing 50 reprints of my paper to key people in the medical profession, the legal profession, and the Church. In addition I wrote to relevant national organisations in the U.K. including the Patients' Association, the Royal College of Nursing, the Department of Health, the Consumer's Council, the Cancer Relief Macmillan Fund, the Association for Palliative Medicine of Great Britain and Ireland, and the Royal College of General Practitioners. Helpful replies from several correspondents indicated a high level of concern about the issue raised.

My remarks were addressed primarily to consultants in palliative medicine and my main concern was to persuade those entrusted with the care of the dying to adopt a more flexible attitude to hydration, to use intravenous or subcutaneous fluids when necessary, to pay due heed to the concerns of relatives and to treat relatives with greater sensitivity.

The published response in professional journals

The attention of the legal profession was drawn to the legal problems posed by sedation without hydration, in a short paper in the Medico-Legal Journal in 1994.[4] I later learnt of the work of John Finnis and others on the concept of murder by omission. A full analysis of this and related issues can be found in "Euthanasia, clinical practice and law" which was published by the Linacre Centre in 1994.[5]

The issues were debated vigorously within the medical profession between 1994 and 1996 and many consultants in palliative medicine took the trouble to respond to my criticism in professional journals. I reviewed their responses in 1996 and took the debate a little further.[6] My contribution to a debate at the Royal College of Physicians in 1997 was later published and proved helpful to members of the general public.[7] Eventually guidelines on the ethical use of artificial hydration in terminally ill patients were published in the European Journal of Palliative Care.[8]

Fainsinger and Bruera in Canada have been leading advocates of the use of subcutaneous hydration in terminally ill cancer patients for many years.[9,10] Their work will be covered in greater detail in a later chapter. Suffice it to say at this stage that their important paper in the Journal of Pain and Symptom Management in 1994 was a timely contribution to the debate. Some years earlier in 1991 they had drawn attention to the value of subcutaneous hydration in symptom control in a specialist journal that is widely available in the UK.[10] Sadly this paper came too late to influence those caring for the patient whose death in 1990 raised my concerns.

The issues were debated in countless hospices throughout the United Kingdom as palliative carers engaged in lively discussion with their colleagues. The ethical use of artificial hydration in terminally ill patients was discussed by the ethics committee of the Association for Palliative Medicine of Great Britain and Ireland under the chairmanship of Dr Ilora Finlay initially, and later under Dr Kilean Dunphy. It was also discussed by the ethics committee of the Royal College of Physicians of London and by the Linacre Centre for Health Care Ethics. It required a lot of detective work on my part to keep in touch with developments that often seemed shrouded in secrecy.

Dunlop, Baines, Sykes and Dame Cicely Saunders from St Christopher's Hospice in London, with Ellershaw, Medical Director of the Marie Curie Centre in Liverpool responded with a paper in the Journal of Medical Ethics.[11] They felt that nutritional support 'may be helpful for a small number of patients who have local disease causing swallowing difficulties but who are not yet dying from widely disseminated endstage cancer, for example those with head and neck cancers'. They agree that there are rare occasions when it is justifiable to give subcutaneous fluids for the sake of the family, but do not recommend the routine use of intravenous or subcutaneous fluids, primarily because of concerns about possible harm in patients with a low serum albumin. They have noticed that 'Patients who are dying of cancer usually give up eating and then stop drinking…' Following on from this they incline to the view that 'hunger is not a feature of the anorexia-cachexia syndrome'. (This medical term is used to describe a combination of loss of appetite and general wasting in terminal cancer patients.) Dunlop *et al* also believe that 'thirst is not associated with decreasing fluid intake in those close to death…' [11] In other words they believe that terminal dehydration is not associated with thirst in cancer patients who are close to death. This is a widely held view among palliative carers, but I do not find it convincing, for reasons that will become apparent. The full text of the paper by Dunlop *et al.* can be found in the next chapter of this book.

Dr Michael Ashby, a Professor of Palliative Care at Monash University, and Brian Stoffell, a bioethicist and Director of the Medical Ethics Unit at Flinders University of South Australia liaised with Dr L Hepburn, Director of the Provincial Bioethics Unit for Queensland, and with Professor Margaret Somerville and the staff of the Centre for Medical Ethics and Law of McGill University, Montreal, Canada. The resulting paper by Ashby and Stoffell was published in the Journal of Medical Ethics in 1995.[12]

Legal aspects were dealt with from an Australian and Canadian viewpoint. The full text of their paper is reprinted in chapter 4 of this book. Ashby and Stoffell amended their framework for palliative care to take account of some of my comments. They acknowledged that -

- "Artificial hydration may be required in the terminal phase to satisfy thirst, or other symptoms due to lack of fluid intake."
- "The emotional needs and ethical views of the patient's family and care givers must be acknowledged…" and…
- "If artificial hydration and nutrition are identified as necessary for comfort by attending staff or family members, and may be effective in achieving the stated aims, then they should not be refused." [12]

An important and challenging paper by Dunphy, Finlay, Rathbone *et al* in the journal Palliative Medicine should be read by all palliative carers who are seriously interested in the hydration debate.[13]

New text books appeared on palliative care

Dr Fiona Randall was given sabbatical leave from her post in the south of England to write a book on palliative care ethics with Professor R S Downie, a moral philosopher based in Glasgow. Little of substance was said about hydration but some useful legal comments were made with advice from Mr J Montgomery of the Faculty of Law, Southampton University. The book, published by Oxford University Press in 1996, provides revealing insight into the thought processes that lead to treatment-limiting decisions in palliative care. A chapter on clinical treatment decisions is prefaced with a quotation that encapsulates the death-orientated approach to palliative care . . . "You do me wrong to take me out o' the grave." (Shakespeare, King Lear, Act 4, Scene 7). However, King Lear had just been woken from a deep sleep when he said this. On coming to his senses he said "You must bear with me. Pray you now, forget and forgive. I am old and foolish." [14]

It is fair to say that there has been an explosion of books on medical ethics and palliative care in recent years, for the ethical use of medical technology and 'end-of-life' decisions are now centre stage. Oxford University Press published another book on palliative care in 1996, edited jointly by a Canadian/British duo, Professor Eduardo Bruera and Dr Irene Higginson. This book included a chapter on hydration. [15]

The British Medical Journal published an excellent series of articles on palliative care from September 1997 onwards. These articles were later published as a book 'The ABC of Palliative Care' in 1998. [16]

The hidden debate in the UK

Behind the scenes a working party was set up to prepare guidelines on the ethical use of artificial hydration in the terminally ill. Dr Fiona Randall, a palliative medicine specialist, chaired a joint working party between the National Council for Hospice and Specialist Palliative Care Services (NCHSPCS) and the ethics committee of the Association for Palliative Medicine of Great Britain and Ireland. Finally in 1997 guidelines on the ethical use of artificial hydration in terminally ill patients and on cardiopulmonary resuscitation were published in the European Journal of Palliative Care. [8] A copy of the guidelines can be found in the Appendix of this book.

The guidelines were prepared by a working party, convened in 1995, in response to my "robust" criticism voiced in the Journal of Medical Ethics. The working party was drawn from the ethics committees of the Association for Palliative Medicine of Great Britain and Ireland and the National Council for Hospice and Specialist Palliative Care Services. In the next two years they took advice from the British Medical Association, the Royal College of Nursing, the Department of Health and the NHS Executive. Advice on specific legal and ethical points was provided by the Centre for Medical Ethics and Law, Kings College London. [17]

Comments by Randall and Downie on the subject of guidelines are of particular interest, bearing in mind that Dr Randall chaired the Joint Working Party that produced the NCHSPCS guidelines of 1997. They state (on page 66 of their book) that "Imposition of certain treatment and care plans by purchasers threatens the whole ethos of palliative care." Later they say "There is a danger . . . that professionals may be tempted to evade legal and moral accountability for individual decisions by claiming that their only responsibility is to follow the guidelines, no matter how inappropriate the resulting course may be for a particular patient... it will require some courage to act contrary to guidelines".[14] Thus it is clear that some palliative medicine physicians resent the imposition of guidelines. Others welcome them and recognise the need to set boundaries.

The chief aim of the guidelines as stated by Dunphy and Randall was "to encourage palliative carers to make patient- centred decisions, unhindered by the prejudice of an uncritical commitment to either an acute model of interventionist care, or indeed, to an overly rigid interpretation of hospice philosophy." [17] The wording of the guidelines was cautious and gave ample room for free interpretation, but the message that hydration must be carefully considered was clear.

Discussion at Conferences in the U.K

The issues raised in the Journal of Medical Ethics were debated at several conferences throughout the UK in subsequent years. Some, but not all of the proceedings were published. Conferences tend to be staging points that mark significant progress or significant dissent. Official conference reports, like the minutes of meetings, tend to be sanitised accounts that reveal only what the writers choose to put on record. The accounts that follow are based on my personal observations and show the trends of thought that prevailed in the medical profession at the time.

1. The Royal College of Physicians of London provided a forum for debate in 1997.

Their Conference on 'Palliative Care in General Medicine' ended with a debate on the management of fluid balance in terminal care. This marked the end of a phase of activity leading up to publication of the ethical guidelines.[8]

The debate was opened by Dr Kilean Dunphy, who found little evidence that rehydration relieves the symptoms of dehydration, including thirst. On the other hand he acknowledged that hydration may be indicated in patients with a raised serum calcium, overtreatment with diuretics, recurrent vomiting, diarrhoea, febrile illnesses and a chronically reduced fluid intake. In fact, he conceded that there are many situations when hydration is needed.

In replying, I drew attention to the dangers of dehydration and referred to the work of Fainsinger and Bruera, who offer subcutaneous fluids to all their patients who are dehydrated or at risk of becoming so. They find that the average duration of use in the terminal phase of life is 14 days. Their experience indicates that about two thirds of the patients in a palliative care unit, especially those who deteriorate slowly, need subcutaneous fluids.[10] I questioned some basic tenets of hospice care and proposed a more life-orientated approach.[7] My key message was that *attention to hydration is not merely an option, it should be a basic part of good medicine and good palliative care.* I warned colleagues that there are times when sedation without hydration seems tantamount to euthanasia.

Discussion was lively! The general conclusion noted in the conference report was that *"careful clinical assessment and diagnosis of every problem is the central premise of palliative care. A blanket policy of artificial hydration or no artificial hydration is ethically indefensible. Each case is unique. Doctors need to respect the individual's previous requests and address the anxieties of relatives.*[18] That statement summarises the position that the profession had reached in the UK in 1997. Points requiring further attention at that stage are shown in Table 1.

Table 1 *Points requiring further attention* [19]

- The practice of sedation without hydration in palliative care is open to misuse.
- When sedation without hydration is considered for any reason a second consultant opinion should be obligatory, for "doctors are as likely as anyone else to make mistakes and err in judgement." [20]
- There should be a confidential inquiry into the use of parenteral sedation in palliative care, and some effective monitoring system.
- There is a need to address the issue of how best to resolve clinical ethical disputes during life. Some forum in which relatives can participate is needed. (see Gillon [2])
- There is a need for research to determine whether thirst really is reduced in patients dying of cancer, and if so, what is the mechanism? If thirst is reduced, such patients, like the healthy elderly, will be at increased risk of dehydration.

2. Conference on Compassionate Care for the Dying. London, March 1998

Two major pro-life organisations- the International Right to Life Federation and the Society for the Protection of Unborn Children (SPUC) held a combined conference in London in 1998. Speakers included Mr Luke Gormally, Dr Jack Willke, Dr Nigel Sykes and others. My account of the proceedings is confined to two talks that were of direct relevance to the hydration debate. Mixed messages were given about double effect. My report is based on my contemporaneous notes.

On intention, hypocrisy and double effect

In a plenary session one speaker Mr Brendon Gerard, took the view that some shortening of life was acceptable if not out of proportion to the good intended. Non-treatment decisions tended to be a consequence of the futility argument and concern about the burden to the patient. He recognised that the double effect principle can be misused and misapplied and said that intention to shorten life is criminal and double effect can be a cover for euthanasia. Another speaker, a Catholic Bishop from the USA referred to comments in the New York Times in 1994, and mentioned that when a certain doctor called a morphine drip 'euthanasia' he was ridiculed. People are worried that concern about double effect will reduce confidence in pain control, he said, so the euthanasia lobby in the USA have been asked to drop this argument. There is a view that where life is worthwhile but burdensome, the end of life may be a benefit, said the Bishop.

On the costs and benefits of palliative care [21]

Dr Nigel Sykes, a British palliative care specialist outlined the support currently available in the United Kingdom. 97% of patients referred to palliative care specialists have advanced cancer- the remaining 3% have motor neurone disease, AIDS, end stage respiratory disease, heart or kidney failure. Specialist care reaches at least 40% of patients at home with cancer, said Dr Sykes. Inpatient care is provided in the hospice network, where the average length of stay is two weeks. 40% of hospice patients go home initially. Hospices also provide day care that may include a hair-do, art therapy, reminiscence and discussion about illness. Hospital based advisory teams support hospital doctors and nurses- a service pioneered at St.Thomas's Hospital.

Home care is provided by Macmillan and Marie Curie nurses- the latter will provide night sitting nurses. Home respite teams of hospice nurses supplement district nurses. Funding for palliative care in 1998 came largely from charitable sources, but 40% came from the National Health Service.[21]

On the subject of pain control

Dr Sykes advised that one should deal with fears and give information, regular follow up and support. Use of the World Health Organisation (WHO) analgesic step-ladder process, whereby analgesic drugs are given starting with the mildest and working up to the strongest as necessary, gives pain relief in 80-90% of patients. Very occasionally sedation is needed. He referred to 'myths about morphine' and stated that if anything it increases life- improved mobility for example can reduce the incidence of pneumonia. Addiction is not an issue said Sykes and this view is confirmed in the literature.[23, 24] He stressed that morphine will not stupefy if carefully titrated i.e. if doses are increased in careful increments until pain is controlled. The limitations of treatment with morphine are constipation, nausea, and non-responsive pains that may arise from nerves or bones, sometimes in relation to movement.

Sykes stated that double effect hardly ever has to be invoked in palliative medicine. That statement may be true if one disregards the fatal effect of drug-induced dehydration- but in my opinion, to do so is intellectually dishonest. As Dunphy and Finlay noted- in a paper that Sykes must surely have seen- 'Dehydration retains the potential to be an important cause of morbidity in seriously ill patients. The onus rests with palliative care physicians to assess the degree of dehydration, and whether this is likely to be contributing to the patient's deteriorating condition...' [13]

On the subject of terminal agitation

Dr Sykes stated that in 10-25% of cases sedation is required briefly and does not shorten life. Then as an afterthought he announced to the assembled audience of professional and lay people- "If you hear that people are being sedated to death, say that it does not happen. If it happens it is bad medicine!" Rightly or wrongly, I formed the opinion that this comment was a direct response to my criticism in the Journal of Medical Ethics. I made a mental note of the remark, but refrained from speaking out on that occasion.

3. The Centre for Bioethics and Public Policy provided a forum for debate in 1998

A Conference on 'Palliative Care - The Way Forward' organised by a Christian ethics think-tank, the Centre for Bioethics and Public Policy (CBPP) in November 1998 was attended by delegates from many walks of life. Dame Cicely Saunders opened the conference with an account of how her pioneering work had developed over the years. Dr John Keown, then lecturer in law from Queen's College Cambridge, spoke about the doctrine of double effect,[25] and I was invited to repeat the paper given at the Royal College of Physicians. Other speakers came from Russia, Czechoslovakia and France and included Judge Christian Byk, former bioethics adviser to the Council of Europe. In due course some of the papers were published by the CBPP.[26]

4. Conference on 'Ethical decisions at the end of life'. RCP. London, March 1999

The Royal College of Physicians of London held another conference on medical ethics in 1998. This was, to some extent, a continuation of the hydration debate. The need for a more sensitive approach to relatives was stressed by Professor Finlay, and there was an interesting panel debate on 'double effect'. Delegates were warned by Penney Lewis, a Lecturer in Law at the Institute of Law and Medical Ethics at King's College in London, that this traditional line of medical defence was unsatisfactory.

A talk on hydration or dehydration in the dying patient given by Dr Ellershaw, revealed areas of difficulty and tension. Many of the old arguments about the benefits of dehydration were reiterated with only passing reference to the work of Fainsinger. Ellershaw acknowledged that artificial hydration should be given for correctable causes of dehydration such as a raised serum calcium or vomiting, but with respect to the use of sedation for uncontrolled pain or agitation, he suggested that sedation rarely prevents patients from drinking enough. In the event of dehydration, artificial hydration should be considered, and psychiatrists involved if need be. The impression was given that syringe drivers are started only in the dying phase, defined by Ellershaw as the last 2 days of life, when the patient is already semi-comatose. The situation should be discussed with the patient and the family, but artificial hydration would rarely be given at this stage. Hydration was only one aspect of care he said.

Thus despite all the papers written on the subject of sedation without hydration, some doctors still try to evade serious discussion of the ethical issues.

During the course of his talk Ellershaw announced that it was "unfair of Dr Craig to suggest that sedation without hydration could be fatal…" Palliative carers were, it seemed, riled by reports of my warning to this effect as given to the RCP in 1997 and reported on the front page of The Times in January 1999.[27] I made my presence known and countered this comment during discussion, leaving delegates in little doubt that prolonged sedation without hydration does occur, and when it occurs it is a matter for grave concern. Delegates included the Official Solicitor and Judge Stephen Tumim, who was at that time, chairing a committee on euthanasia. My dejection at the lack of progress and the intransigence of some palliative carers was tempered by pleasure, for sitting at the back of the hall I could see a flutter of blue, like kingfisher wings. These represented 200 complimentary copies of Ethics and Medicine in its distinctive blue cover containing relevant papers, made available to conference delegates with the permission of the Academic Registrar of the College and the generosity of the publisher Paternoster Publishing, UK. The take-up was encouraging!

5. *Debate at the Palliative Care Congress at Warwick in 2000*

In 2000 I was invited to take part in a 'spontaneous' panel discussion on the terminal care of the dying at the Palliative Care Congress in Warwick, England. The 'Medical Treatment (prevention of Euthanasia) Bill' was about to be introduced in the House of Commons and palliative carers were worried. The Bill was drawn up 'to prohibit the withdrawal or withholding of medical treatment, or the withdrawal or withholding of sustenance, with the intention of causing the death of a patient...' It was an attempt to give legal protection to patients such as elderly stroke patients and others, whose lives can be prolonged by measures such as tube feeding. Sadly palliative carers were not unduly concerned about the fate of such patients, for their main concern was with the dying. Towards the end of the session one of the panel, Dr Rachel Burman, who was at that time the chairperson of the ethics committee of the Association for Palliative Medicine of Great Britain and Ireland, read out a prepared statement about the Bill. As delegates were leaving the hall, one of them- Professor Michael Richards, a palliative carer with a government position as the 'Cancer Tsar'- came up to Dr Burman and was handed the prepared statement. No doubt that statement was taken post haste to the Department of Health. The Bill was not supported by the medical establishment or by the Government, and failed, by a narrow margin, to get through Parliament.

Palliative carers fear any legislation that might restrict their freedom in the care of the dying. Yet in doing so they limit the degree of legal protection that can be given to chronically ill patients whose lives can be prolonged, sometimes for years, by measures such as tube feeding. Skill in the care of terminally ill cancer patients does not necessarily qualify a person to advise members of parliament on the care of patients with strokes and dementia, for their medical conditions and needs are entirely different. Yet palliative carers have a strong influence in political circles in the United Kingdom. Those in a position of influence should ensure that they take the best interests of all patients to heart.

The euthanasia question

Palliative carers are naturally concerned to refute any suggestion that taints the hospice movement with even a hint of euthanasia, but taken to extremes this attitude makes it extremely difficult to tackle problems honestly when they occur. A euthanasia working party, chaired by Judge Stephen Tumim was set up in 1998 under the auspices of the Royal College of Physicians and the Royal College of General Practitioners. The membership was not divulged at the time. Their terms of reference as set out in a press statement dated 7th October 1998 were:

- To identify to the RCP/RCGP the kinds of conduct which constitute euthanasia, and advise how far they can be justified on moral grounds.
- To describe and evaluate the current situation and consider the implications of change.
- To advise on the part health professionals should play in public debate and policy making.

The last aim was rather like shutting the stable door after the horse had bolted! Doctors who favour a change in the law are already actively promoting their aims in public, and have tried to turn the issue of sedation without hydration to their advantage. In general however, euthanasia is not a subject that the medical profession like to discuss, as was evident at the RCP Conference in March 1999. Many doctors rightly consider that active euthanasia should have no place in medicine.

Reporting in 2001 the Tumim Committee said 'It is clear that the intention behind a predominantly therapeutic decision, in contrast to its foreseen outcome, is a central issue for further debate within the profession and within society.' [28]

Perhaps if people thought of parenteral sedation as a potentially lethal injection, given slowly over a matter of days, the ethical and legal issues would become clearer. The Voluntary Euthanasia Society have been quick to grasp the fact that prolonged sedation without hydration can cause death just as surely as a lethal injection.

If palliative carers are to maintain their position of trust as opponents of euthanasia it is essential for them to pay more heed to hydration in the terminally ill.

International aspects of the debate

The debate spread around the world through the *Journal of Medical Ethics* from England and Canada, to the USA, Australia and Japan. A paper by Morita and colleagues in Japan, published in an American journal in June 1999,[29] reached me promptly via a colleague in Wales! I thank all those who, through such acts of courtesy, have eased my task over the years.

My view of the debate is inevitably biased towards events in the United Kingdom, for that was my personal sphere of activity. A local or national approach may seem parochial to international jet-setting doctors, but small is beautiful. It is essential to remember that human society is varied. National characteristics and culture remain extremely important, and we all have to work through our national institutions.

International communication of medical advances is of course essential, and we need cross-fertilisation of ideas. We also need to learn from other people's mistakes, for what seems ethical and appropriate in one country may not be applicable in another. Political and legal aspects of the debate will vary from country to country, depending on prevailing conditions and laws. For all these reasons, I have not attempted to review the world-wide situation in any detail in this book.

My experience has shown that it is still possible for an individual, supported by a highly respected medical journal to influence events.

References and notes

1. Craig G M. On withholding nutrition and hydration in the terminally ill. Has palliative medicine gone too far ? *Journal of Medical Ethics* 1994; **20**: 139-141.
2. Gillon R. (editorial). Palliative care ethics: non-provision of artificial nutrition and hydration to terminally ill sedated patients. *Journal of medical ethics* 1994. **20**: 131-2, 187.
3. Wilkes E. On withholding nutrition and hydration in the terminally ill: has palliative medicine gone too far? A commentary. *Journal of Medical Ethics* 1994; **20**: 144-5.
4. Craig G M. Is sedation without hydration or nourishment in terminal care lawful? *Medico-Legal Journal* 1994; **62**: 198-201.

5. Euthanasia, clinical practice and the law. Ed. Luke Gormally. *The Linacre Centre for Health Care Ethics*. 1994.
6. Craig G M. On withholding artificial hydration and nutrition from terminally ill sedated patients. The debate continues. *Journal of Medical Ethics* 1996; **22**: 147-153.
7. Craig G M. Palliative care from the perspective of a consultant geriatrician. The dangers of withholding hydration. *Ethics and Medicine* 1999; **15;1** 15-19.
8. Artificial hydration (AH) for people who are terminally ill. *European Journal of Palliative Care* 1997; **4**: 124. Copyright remains with the National Council for Hospice and Specialist Palliative Care Services, London.
9. Fainsinger R L, MacEarchern T, Miller M J. *et al.* The use of hypodermoclysis for rehydration in terminally ill cancer patients. *Journal of Pain and Symptom Management* 1994; **9**: 198-302.
10. Fainsinger R. Bruera L. Hypodermoclysis (HDC) for symptom control vs. the Edmonton Injector (EI). *Journal of Palliative Care* 1991; **7**: 5-8.
11. Dunlop R, Ellershaw J E, Baines M J, Sykes N, Saunders C. On withholding nutrition and hydration in the terminally ill: has palliative medicine gone too far? *A* reply . *Journal of Medical Ethics 1995*. **21**: 141-3.
12. Ashby M. and Stofell B. Artificial hydration and alimentation at the end of life: a reply to Craig. *Journal of Medical Ethics* 1995; **21**: 135-40.
13. Dunphy K, Finlay I, Rathbone G, Gilbert J, Hick F. Rehydration in palliative and terminal care: if not why not? *Palliative Medicine* 1995; **9**: 221-8.
14. Randall F and Downie R S. Palliative Care Ethics 1996; Oxford University Press.
15. MacDonald N, Fainsinger R. Indications and ethical considerations in the hydration of patients with advanced cancer. In Bruera E. and Higginson I eds. Cachexia-anorexia in cancer patients. Oxford. Oxford University Press 1996; p 94-109.
16. The ABC of Palliative Care, BMJ Books 1998.
17. Dunphy K and Randall F. Ethical decision making in palliative care. *European Journal of Palliative Care* 1997; **4:** 126-128.
18. Conference report. Journal of the Royal College of Physicians of London 1997; **31**: 695-699.
19. Craig G M. (letter) Palliative care in general medicine. *Journal of the Royal College of Physicians of London* 1998. **32**: 83.
20. Report into the Committee of Inquiry into South Ockendon Hospital, London. *HMSO* 1974.
21. For further information about funding and other issues see "New Themes in Palliative Care." Ed. Clark D, Hockley J and Ahmedzai S. *Open University Press 1997*
22. For a recent review see Sykes N and Thoms A. The use of opioids and sedatives at the end of life. *The Lancet* 2003; **4;** 312-318
23. Angell M. "The quality of mercy" *New England Journal of Medicine* 1982; **306**: 99. quoted by SPUC in March 1998.
24. Scott J. "Fear and false promises: the challenge of pain in the terminally ill." In Ian Gentles, Euthanasia and Assisted Suicide: The Current Debate. *Stoddart*: Toronto 1995 p 52. quoted by SPUC March 1998.

25. Keown J. 'Double effect' and Palliative Care: A legal and ethical outline. *Ethics and Medicine* 1999; **15**: 53-54.
26. Palliative Care: The Way Forward. CBPP, 53 Romney Street, London SW1P 3RF. 1998.
27. Horsnell M. Police check for "backdoor euthanasia." *The Times*, London, January 6th 1999, page 1.
28. Medical treatment at the end of life. A position statement. *Clinical Medicine* 2001; **1:** 115-117.
29. Morita T, Tsunoda J, Inoue S, Chihara S. Perceptions and decision-making on rehydration of terminally ill cancer patients and family members. *American Journal of Hospice and Palliative Care* 1999; **16**: 509-516.

Chapter 4

Traditional Palliative Carers
Defend Their Position

On withholding nutrition and hydration in the terminally ill: has palliative medicine gone too far? A reply.

R.J. Dunlop, J.E. Ellershaw, M.J. Baines, N. Sykes and C.M. Saunders. Journal of Medical Ethics. 1995: 21:141-143. © BMJ Publishing Group. Reprinted with permission.

Abstract

Patients who are dying of cancer usually give up eating and then stop drinking. This raises ethical dilemmas about providing nutritional support and fluid replacement. The decision-making process should be based on a knowledge of the risks and benefits of giving or withholding treatments. There is no clear evidence that increased nutritional support of fluid therapy alters comfort, mental status or survival of patients who are dying. Rarely subcutanenous fluid administration in the dying patient may be justified if the family remain distressed despite due consideration of the lack of medical benefit versus the risks. Some cancer patients who are not imminently dying become dehydrated from reversible conditions such as hypercalcaemia. This may mimic the effects of advanced cancer. These conditions should be sought and fluid replacement therapy should be given along with the specific treatments for the condition.

The issues surrounding the management of fluid and nutritional status in the terminally ill were brought sharply into focus by Dr Craig.[1] She rightly pointed out the dangers of automatically withholding fluid replacement therapy. Palliative care never has been, and never should be, an excuse for bad medicine. The need for careful clinical assessment and diagnosis of every problem is a central premise of palliative care. Reversible conditions such as hypercalcaemia may cause dehydration in patients who are not imminently dying. If rehydration is not carried out the patient will deteriorate rapidly. The gaunt appearance and altered state will mimic the effects of advanced cancer.

It is important to distinguish those patients for whom fluid replacement is medically indicated. A distinction can often be made on clinical grounds. Dying patients have a longer history (weeks or months) of gradual deterioration with increasing weakness, fatigue, weight loss and drowsiness. Dehydration will cause more rapid deterioration, usually over days, in the setting of a precipitating cause, suggested by the history (for example, polyuria, polydipsia with hypercalcaemia,or vomiting from bowel obstruction), clinical examination and appropriate laboratory findings. The acute change will cause considerable distress both to the patient and the family. Such distress should be used as a further prompt to search for a reversible problem. It should be born in mind that some people deny the previous history of gradual decline and then 'suddenly' become distressed when the patient finally stops swallowing. When there is doubt, a therapeutic trial of fluids and other appropriate treatments may well be warranted so long as the wishes of the patient are not contravened.

On the other hand, most terminally ill patients reach a point during their gradual physical decline when they first stop eating and then subsequently stop drinking. This occurs even in patients who are not taking medications and as Dr Craig pointed out, this situation arouses considerable distress for relatives. Dr Gillon discussed the principles which should be followed when conflict arises between proxies and staff.[2] However, conflict may be prevented by anticipatory dialogue based on the evidence for the risks and benefits of giving versus withholding treatment.

Nutritional support should be considered as a separate issue from dehydration. The administration of conventional dextrose solutions via peripheral veins does not constitute nutritional support. This can only be achieved by enteral feeding (nasogastric tube or gastrostomy) or by parenteral administration into a central vein. Although patients with advanced cancer appear to be malnourished, the metabolic abnormalities are quite different from starvation in an otherwise healthy person. There is no evidence that in patients with advanced cancer, aggressive nutritional support, either enteral or parenteral, prolongs life or even significantly alters the metabolic abnormalities.[3] Indeed there is evidence that cancer growth may be accelerated, thereby increasing local symptoms from the cancer.[4] Nutritional support may be helpful for the small number of patients who have local disease causing swallowing difficulties but who are not yet dying from disseminated endstage cancer, for example, those with head and neck cancers.

Dehydration results from an intake of water below the minimum required to maintain homeostasis. In someone who is otherwise healthy, the symptoms are thirst, dry mouth, headache, fatigue, then cognitive impairment followed by sequelae described by Dr Craig: circulatory collapse, renal failure, anuria and death. The first clue suggesting that the situation in cancer patients is not equivalent to acute dehydration came from clinical observations in dying patients who were not taking any medications and who did not have correctable causes for their dehydration. In such patients systemic symptoms such as fatigue and drowsiness usually precede the cessation of fluid intake by several days or weeks. Even though these patients may be very drowsy at the time they stop drinking, they can rouse and respond to questions from family for example.

Analysis of blood and urine chemistry in terminally ill patients has failed to disclose evidence of the expected changes from dehydration.[5,6] In a recent prospective study of dying cancer patients (median time to death, two days) the symptoms of dry mouth were not correlated with the level of hydration.[6] These findings support the work of Burge who investigated dehydration symptoms in 51 cancer patients with an estimated prognosis of less than 6 weeks. He found no significant association between biochemical markers of dehydration (serum osmolality, urea, sodium) and the symptom of thirst.[7] Therefore giving additional fluid to dying patients in order to alleviate the symptoms of dry mouth and thirst may well be futile.

In the same way that hunger is not a feature of the anorexia-cachexia syndrome, thirst is not associated with decreasing fluid intake in those close to death. It is possible that the normal homeostatic mechanisms controlling fluid intake and fluid balance are altered in the dying process. Further evidence for this hypothesis derives from studies of patients given fluids intravenously. Waller *et al* compared 55 patients treated with oral fluids with 13 patients who received IV fluids.[8] They found no difference in the biochemical parameters and state of consciousness between the two groups.

It seems reasonable to conclude from these observations that nutritional or fluid supplementation cannot be automatically justified on medical grounds for patients dying of advanced cancer. Is fluid harmful? To our knowledge, no studies have demonstrated any adverse effects from fluid therapy. Intravenous fluids can pose a problem to patient comfort if the arm needs splinting. This can be overcome by using the subcutaneous route. Terminally ill patients have lower albumin levels [6] which may cause problems when crystalloid solutions are administered. Albumin is the plasma protein which is largely responsible for maintaining colloid osmotic pressure. This pressure counteracts the forces which tend to move fluid out of blood vessels. The authors have seen patients develop pulmonary oedema, rapidly increasing ascites, and unsightly peripheral oedema involving conjunctivae and the hands when given intravenous fluids in acute hospital wards, particularly if the serum albumin is below 26 g/l.

Dr Craig drew attention to the use of sedation in terminal care. Once again, a careful history and examination is necessary to distinguish terminal agitation from a reversible problem in someone who is not actually dying. Terminal agitation must be treated aggressively, otherwise the distress of the patient will become extreme. Even when incremental doses of sedatives are given, it is rarely possible to achieve a balance between relief of agitation and alertness. All palliative carers would echo the experience of Wilkes who described the problems of trying to reduce the dose of sedatives when the patient is settled.[9]

When sedation is required in a patient who is not actually dying, we rarely find that it is necessary to render the patient unconscious. Nursing staff can still feed the patient and maintain hydration. The dose of tranquillisers is always reduced to the lowest level necessary to control the symptoms. We would seek the advice of a psychiatrist in treating such cases.

Given that there is no clear evidence of symptomatic benefit from nutritional or fluid therapy in cancer patients who are dying and that there is potential harm if there is severe hypoalbuminaemia, we do not recommend the routine use of intravenous or subcutaneous fluids. When discussing these issues with a family, it is important not to argue from some philosophical standpoint, but it is important to present the facts carefully. On most occasions, families will be reassured and their sense of helplessness can be assuaged by encouraging them to perform mouth care. Some families (particularly from some cultural and religious backgrounds) may not be satisfied. In these circumstances, so long as no contrary opinion has been expressed by the patient, we give subcutaneous fluids for the sake of the family. This situation only arises two to three times per 1,000 admissions per year at St Christopher's Hospice. The volume is kept to no more than one litre per 24 hours to avoid overload. The use of a local anaesthetic cream will prevent pain from the cannula insertion. The infusion is usually given overnight; the subcutaneous line is capped and left in-situ during the day so that the patient is not subjected to multiple needle pricks. By giving the infusion intermittently, it is easier for the family to make the decision to discontinue therapy.

R J Dunlop, FRACP is Medical Director of St Christopher's Hospice. J E Ellershaw, MRCP, is Medical Director of the Liverpool Marie Curie Centre. M J Baines, OBE, MRCP, is Consultant Physician at St Christopher's Hospice. N Sykes, MA, MRCGP, is also Consultant Physician at St Christopher's Hospice, and C M Saunders, OM, DBE, FRCP, is Chairman of St Christopher's Hospice.

References

1. Craig. G M. On withholding nutrition and hydration in the terminally ill: has palliative medicine gone too far? *Journal of Medical Ethics* 1994; 20: 139-143.
2. Gillon R. Palliative care ethics: non-provision of artificial nutrition and hydration to terminally ill sedated patients. *Journal of Medical Ethics* 1994; 20: 131-132,187.
3. Brennan M F. Total parenteral nutrition in the cancer patient. *New England Journal of Medicine* 1981; 305: 373-375.
4. Rice M I, Van Rij A M. Parenteral nutrition and tumour growth in the patient with complicated abdominal cancer. *Australia and New Zealand journal of surgery* 1887; 57: 375-379.
5. Oliver D. Terminal dehydration. *Lancet* 1984; 2: 631.
6. Ellershaw J E, Sutcliffe J M, Saunders C M. Dehydration and the dying patient. *Journal of Pain and Symptom Management* (in press).
7. Burge F I. Dehydration symptoms of palliative care cancer patients. *Journal of Pain and Symptom Management* 1993; 8,7:454-464.
8. Waller A, Adunski A, Hershkowitz M. Terminal dehydration and intravenous fluids. *Lancet* 1991; 337: 745.
9. Wilkes E. On withholding nutrition and hydration in the terminally ill: has palliative medicine gone too far? A commentary. *Journal of Medical Ethics* 1994; 20: 144-145.

Dehydration and the dying patient

Ellershaw JE. Sutcliffe J. Saunders CM. Journal of Pain and Symptom Management 1995; 10: 192-197.

Review and comments by Craig

This oft-cited paper was in press (see reference 6 above) when the response by Dunlop, Ellershaw, Baines *et al* was published in the Journal of Medical Ethics. The authors referred to discussion in the literature about 'the appropriateness of withholding or withdrawing artificial fluid therapy (intravenous, subcutaneous, nasogastric or rectal) in the dying patient,' but made no mention of the debate in the Journal of Medical Ethics in 1994, choosing instead to refer to earlier work on the topic.

Ellershaw, Sutcliffe and Saunders were unhappy about the use of the phrase 'terminal dehydration' in the dying as they felt that the term was 'emotionally charged and may perpetuate the practice of hydrating dying patients without any scientific evidence to support this treatment.' They then set out to try to assess the relationship between biochemical dehydration and some common symptoms in the dying.

The authors described a study undertaken at St Christopher's Hospice, London. An attempt was made to correlate respiratory tract secretions, thirst and symptoms of a dry mouth in 82 dying patients, with the level of dehydration as judged by biochemical analysis of serum samples. The median time from entry into the study and death was two days. All subjects had malignant disease and died without artificial fluid therapy, according to traditional hospice practice. Statistical analysis of the results was undertaken by Fiona Reed of King's College Hospital, London.

Of the 82 subjects studied, 19 (23%) had carcinoma of the lung- a group in which death is often sudden and not associated with progressive dehydration according to Fainsinger *et al.* (Journal of Pain and Symptom Management 1994; 9: 298-302). In addition it is well known that patients with carcinoma of the lung may have inappropriate secretion of anti-diuretic hormone with abnormal fluid retention associated with low serum sodium and abnormally low plasma osmolality levels. This confounding factor was not considered by the authors, but could have influenced overall results. 25% of subjects studied had a plasma osmolality within the normal range of 274-295 mOsm/kg. The overall mean level was a little raised at 298.6 mOsm/kg. and the range was wide being between 259 and 418 mOsm/kg. Thus some patients had significantly high or significantly low plasma osmolality levels. Those with abnormally low levels would be expected to have reduced thirst sensation.

For purposes of statistical analysis patients were divided into two groups- those without biochemical dehydration (Group A) and those with biochemical dehydration (Group B). Dehydration was excluded if the serum osmolality was within the normal range, the serum creatinine (a measure of renal function) was less than 130 (normal range 60-120 umol/l) and the blood urea was less than 12 mmol/l. (normal 2.5-6.5). Thus somewhat elevated levels of creatinine and urea were accepted as 'normal'. On this basis 21 subjects (group A) were considered to have no dehydration, and the rest (group B) were considered to be dehydrated. It is not clear to which group patients with a low osmolality were allocated.

All subjects in group A developed respiratory tract secretions (as judged by audible sounds at the bedside) but 11% of group B did not. These trends were not statistically significant.

Barely a quarter of the patients studied could reply to questions, but of those who could 87% complained of a dry mouth (5 in group A and 15 in group B) and 83% complained of thirst (6 in group A and 13 in group B). A high percentage of this small group of responsive patients were on drugs known to cause a dry mouth. On the basis of these results the authors concluded that 'the subjective sensation of thirst is evidently not solely dependent on the level of hydration....therefore giving patients artificial hydration to relieve a dry mouth may be futile...' However in my view an alternative interpretation could be argued, for the published data shows that far more patients complained of a dry mouth and thirst in group B, than in group A. The authors however chose to interpret their results in a way that shored up traditional hospice practice for while recognising the need for further research, they concluded that 'Thirst may be related to the sensation of dry mouth and not centrally mediated through dehydration. The use of artificial hydration to relieve these symptoms may, therefore be futile.'

Acknowledgement

Information and quotations from *"Dehydration and the dying patient"* by Ellershaw *J E, Sutcliffe J and Saunders C M are reprinted from the Journal of Pain and Symptom Management 1995; 10; 192-197 with permission from the US Cancer Pain Relief Committee.*

Published correspondence

Dr Stone and Dr Phillips writing in the correspondence columns of the Journal of Medical Ethics in 1995 claimed that many of my fears were misplaced. I countered this comment through the editor, in a letter that revealed the attitudes of several key people in palliative medicine in the United Kingdom, as expressed to me in personal correspondence. Dame Cicely Saunders and Dr Ilora Finlay were both enthusiastic about the use of subcutaneous fluids. My reply to Stone and Phillips ran as follows-

Nutrition, dehydration and the terminally ill. (Letter)

Reprinted from the Journal of Medical Ethics 1995; 21: 184-185, with permission.

Sir- Your correspondents Dr Stone and Dr Phillips have made some comments on my paper, which was critical of some aspects of palliative medicine (i). They claim that many of my fears were misplaced 'because of a misunderstanding of current practice in palliative medicine.' My paper was the outcome of close observation of current practice, profound concern about what I observed, and examination of the relevant literature up to 1992.

Dr Stone and Dr Phillips concede that when patients are symptomatic, i.e. they complain of thirst but cannot swallow, palliative care physicians will supply fluids artificially. They outline several situations where fluids would not be given, and stray widely from the central theme of my paper which was the need for artificial hydration when a person is rendered incapable of swallowing by sedation. I am not talking about 'a certain amount of physiological dehydration' in the dying process, but of gross iatrogenic dehydration. As I pointed out if sedation is continued without hydration death from dehydration will be inevitable, whatever the underlying pathology, within about seven days. Of course death from natural causes may occur first, but the longer the interval between sedation and death, the greater will be the dehydration element in the aetiology.

Your correspondents refer to a letter written by Waller *et al* (ii) which purports to show that in dying patients the level of consciousness is not affected by the use or non-use of intravenous (IV) fluids. The data does not stand up to scrutiny. Waller measured some biochemical parameters and the level of consciousness in 68 cancer patients during the last 48 hours of life. It is possible to calculate from the information given that the blood urea of all 68 patients at some stage (presumably on admission) was 21.64 mmol/l. Thirteen patients received IV fluids in unspecified amounts, for unspecified lengths of time, either because they were receiving them on transfer, or after family requests. The initial blood urea results in this sub-group of patients are not given. We are told that the mean blood urea- presumably at the end of the study- did not differ in those given, or not given IV fluids, the values being 50.9 and 54.5 mmol/l. Serum sodium was significantly lower in the treated than the untreated group. Level of consciousness did not correlate with the use or non-use of IV fluids but it did correlate with the serum sodium concentration. Serum potassium levels were dangerously high (mean 7.25 mmol/l) in 31 out of 68 patients. This unsatisfactory study does not demonstrate that 'there is a difference between the acute and the dying patient' as Drs Stone and Phillips claim. The high blood urea in the 'treated' group suggests that rehydration was inadequate. The report confirms that many patients in a palliative care setting have no treatment, or inadequate treatment for severe dehydration and electrolyte imbalance.

Drs Stone and Phillips argue that a patient who is sedated for delirium may become dehydrated more slowly than an unsedated delirious person. This may be true but the evidence is lacking. What is certain is that with the passage of time fatal dehydration will occur in both situations unless adequate amounts of fluid are given. Your correspondents state that 'the principal reason that a drip is not sited in palliative care is futility', but opinions as to what is futile and what is not can vary widely. In cases of doubt, especially where survival outcome is uncertain, the balance should be weighted in favour of prolonging life. Relatives' views should be carefully heeded, if the symptoms of pathological grief and post-traumatic stress are to be avoided.

Your correspondents finally retreat behind a wall of conventional jargon, accusing me of 'medicalising dying'. This does not move the debate forward. My concern is about medicalising dying in a literal sense- that is by the giving of medication that may hasten death, if side effects are ignored.

May I assure Drs Stone and Phillips that recent work indicates that patients dying at home who need sedation, do not necessarily have to be admitted for IV fluids. Dame Cicely Saunders is 'finding a real use in the subcutaneous route which can be used at home…(iii).

The ethics committee of the Association for Palliative Medicine discussed the issues raised in my paper, including the need to ensure that the wishes of the family are not disregarded by any global policy of a unit, and the need to look at hydration as a specific patient need. I hope that they will publish a detailed response. Dr Ilora Finlay, the chairperson, expressing her personal opinion, wrote: 'I would agree whole-heartedly that individual assessments must be made, and that rehydration can provide effective symptomatic relief as well as being life-prolonging. The ease with which subcutaneous fluids can be given means that venous access is not a prerequisite.' (iv)

Professor Hanks, writing in his capacity as Director of the Cancer Relief Macmillan Fund said ' The subject raised by your paper concerns a frequent therapeutic dilemma in palliative care practice. The overriding principle in dealing with it must be to tailor the management to the individual patient. Thus in some patients intervention with intravenous or subcutaneous fluids is certainly indicated, whereas for others this is an inappropriate course. I am sure that a blanket policy is wrong....' (v). Hanks did not address the profound ethical issues.

The House of Lords Select Committee on Medical Ethics discussed the issue of nutrition and hydration in the terminally ill in relation to the Bland case, but the principles have wider application. They made it clear that it should be unnecessary to consider the withdrawal (or non-introduction) of nutrition or hydration except in circumstances where its administration is in itself a burden to the patient (vi). Legal aspects remain unresolved (vii). Further debate is needed.

References

i.   Craig G M. On withholding nutrition and hydration in the terminally ill: has palliative medicine gone too far? *Journal of medical ethics* 1994; 20:139-143.
ii. Waller A, Adunski A, Hershkowitz M. Terminal dehydration and intravenous fluids (letter) *Lancet* 1991; 337:745.
iii. Saunders C. Personal communication 1994 Oct.
iv. Finlay I. Personal communication 1994 Nov.
v.   Hanks G W. Personal communication Dec 1994.
vi. *House of Lords Select Committee on Medical Ethics Report*. London: *HMSO,* 1994: paras 251-257: Treatment limiting decisions.
vii. Craig GM. Is sedation without hydration or nourishment in palliative care lawful? *Medico-legal journal* 1994; 62: 198-201.

Artificial hydration and alimentation at the end of life: a reply to Craig

Michael Ashby and Brian Stoffell.
Royal Adelaide Hospital and Mary Potter Hospice, and Flinders Medical Centre respectively, Australia.
Journal of Medical Ethics 1995; **21**:135-140. © BMJ Publishing Group.

Abstract

Dr Gillian Craig [1] has argued that palliative medicine services have tended to adopt a policy of sedation without hydration, which under certain circumstances may be medically inappropriate, causative of death and distressing to family and friends. We welcome this opportunity to defend, with an important modification, the approach we proposed without substantive background argument in our original article [2]. We maintain that slowing and eventual cessation of oral intake is a normal part of the natural dying process, that artificial hydration and alimentation (AHA) are not justified unless thirst or hunger are present and cannot be relieved by other means, but food and fluids for (natural) oral consumption should never be 'withdrawn'. The intention of this practice is not to alter the timing of an inevitable death, and sedation is not used, as has been alleged, to mask the effects of dehydration and starvation. The artificial provision of hydration and alimentation is now widely accepted as medical treatment. We believe that arguments that it is not have led to confusion as to whether non-provision or withdrawal of AHA constitutes a cause of death in law. Arguments that it is such a cause appear to be tenuously based on an extraordinary/ordinary categorisation of treatments by Kelly [3] which has subsequently been interpreted as prescriptive in a way quite inconsistent with the Catholic moral tradition from which the distinction is derived. The focus of ethical discourse on decisions at the end of life should be shifted to an analysis of care, needs, proportionality of medical interventions, and processes of communication.

Introduction

Dr Gillian Craig has raised what she sees as serious concerns about the ethical and legal aspects of the practice of palliative medicine, with particular regard to the non-provision of artificial hydration and alimentation (AHA). We will argue that the ethical reasoning which we have developed to describe our practice of palliative care can accommodate Dr Craig's concerns.[2] The sensitivities and consultative process of negotiation which she articulates are well heard, and we believe are already embodied in contemporary palliative care practice.

There is a broad consensus on aims and ethics of palliative care, and an internationally agreed WHO definition,[4] although some diversity of clinical practice and ethical argument has emerged, particularly with regard to the relationship between palliative care and euthanasia.[5,6] This article is written from the perspective of an inpatient hospice unit which functions as the acute/ crisis intervention facility for a comprehensive palliative-care network (hospice, hospital, home). There are no set policies about who may be admitted, and there is no arbitrary requirement for any therapeutic intervention to be stopped prior to admission. Many patients, particularly those who are young, or have haematological malignancies or AIDS, are in real need of hospice care for symptom control, respite or terminal care. However, they are not yet ready to stop chemotherapy, blood transfusions, antibiotics or other so-called 'active' treatments with palliative intent, and AHA would certainly come into this category in our institution. A gradual process of negotiation will allow the cessation, or non-initiation of treatment as the person's condition deteriorates. We agree that abrupt revision of treatment goals, particularly without adequate consultation of patient, family and staff will lead to anger and disharmony which may have lasting adverse consequences. Consequently communication with these persons is required, but it does not mean that the patient is treated in order to comfort the relatives. The issues raised by Dr Craig are discussed under two main headings: clinical, and ethical/legal.

Clinical

Dr Craig acknowledges the high public esteem for hospice and palliative care but goes on to state that 'some doctors have reservations'. The grounds for these are that there is a danger of patients being labelled as 'terminal' by the therapeutically inactive (palliative care) doctor. They may then be denied life-saving medical treatment which would be administered in the same situation by a treatment-orientated physician, perhaps for a wholly or partially reversible condition which has been misdiagnosed. Wilkes acknowledges that this is a real but rare eventuality, which does not occur more than a few times in a professional life time of palliative care practice,[7] and probably no more so than in any other domain of medical practice. Dr Craig cites two case histories where patients were assessed as dying, but were rehydrated and survived. These constitute poor evidence for mistaken or possibly neglectful assessment in palliative care, even if the patients had been seen by a palliative care service (which is not stated). Careful clinical assessment is a *sine qua non* for any medical endeavour, and certainly before entry into any therapeutic model or protocol, although it is, of course, not infallible. When used to judge the robustness of the ethics of palliative care, these cases might at best fall into the category of hard cases which may be mobilised to undermine any approach. It is not suggested that cholycystectomy be banned because occasionally it is performed inappropriately. Many policies and probably most procedures or interventions in the medical context are dangerous if employed 'without due care and thought'. In our service patients from the main teaching hospital which we serve are accompanied by their notes and we insist on fuller clinical information than some referring doctors think is really necessary for palliative care.

Three phases

Dr Craig quotes from an article in which we described an approach based on three phases of a life-threatening incurable illness: curative, palliative and terminal, with different aims and levels of treatment-related morbidity being acceptable in each phase.[2] A similar approach has been described for patients with cancer, for the purpose of making not for resuscitation orders.[8] We stated that in the terminal phase 'no form of artificial hydration or alimentation is undertaken, all measures not required for comfort are withdrawn, and no treatment-related toxicity is acceptable'.[8]

The framework we proposed was not intended to be a rigid and arbitrary 'policy', and we would not make a virtue of death without artificial hydration (in particular), as in some situations it might even be necessary for comfort right up until the time of death. We agreed that our model is ambiguous as presently worded, and should be amended by the addition of the following: '…unless the effects of this are less than the benefits achieved by the treatment. For example artificial hydration may be required in the terminal phase to satisfy thirst or other symptoms attributable to lack of fluid intake.'

Thus we give 'comfort measures' priority, including or excluding AHA as may be the case. It is further stated by Dr Craig that in the last few days of life the lack of food or drink will not contribute to death and artificial hydration would not be appropriate, which is our point entirely.

Important review

It is not usual 'policy' in hospices to sedate patients in order to mask any proposed unpleasant effects of dehydration. Rather sedation is administered when it is needed to alleviate suffering caused by acute organic brain syndromes (particularly where the underlying cause cannot be identified or reversed) and emotional distress for which other non-medical interventions have failed. It is possibly true that sedation may hasten the actual time at which relatively imminent death will occur. But it is not deemed necessary to hydrate sedated patients during the dying process when they are unable to maintain oral intake, as it makes no sense to attempt to treat a transiently reversible component of their overall dying process. Fainsinger and Bruera [9] have undertaken an important review of the clinical arguments for and against hydration, and it is clear that there is more to learn about the physiology and clinical practice in this area of care. Dehydration can be a contributory cause of an organic brain syndrome, but these are usually multifactorial and in our experience rehydration alone rarely improves cognitive function in dying patients. It is also stated that staff in hospices would be more familiar with drips if they used them more often, and that it is this lack of practice that prejudices them against their use. In our hospice all staff are acute-care trained, and are therefore able to deliver whatever level of medical technology is required in the circumstances to maintain comfort (for example, spinal analgesia, venting gastrostomy, central venous lines, etc). They are always eager to learn new techniques which might benefit their patients. Subcutaneous fluid infusion (hypodermoclysis) has gained considerable acceptance as a means of providing fluids in palliative care.[10] This hopefully obviates the need for the practice, described by Wilkes, of infusing tap water into the rectum, especially if this practice is instituted to appease relatives.[7]

In our view Dr Craig's real concerns are ethical and legal rather than clinical, and are based on a belief that medicine has a duty always to prevent death. This preoccupation about 'buying time' suggests a belief that doctors are responsible for death unless they do all possible to sustain life in all circumstances, a situation that Callaghan calls 'technological brinkmanship': 'doctors still do not, as a rule, talk comfortably and directly with patients about death. ... A worry about malpractice, a zest for technology, a deep-seated moral belief in the need to prolong life, and the pressure of families and others often lead to overtreatment and an excessive reliance on technology'.[11]

Such an approach may have unfortunate consequences for medical practice, and is in part responsible for the difficulties which many doctors experience with appropriate treatment abatement for dying people. If the care of dying people is to improve in all its settings, we need to try and address the issue of non-provision of AHA as a cause of death, which was raised by Dr Craig as there appears to be considerable confusion both within the medical and nursing professions, and also for many members of the public.

Ethical and legal

There is now a broad consensus that AHA should be regarded as medical treatment,[12] and Beauchamp and Childress refer unequivocally to medically administered nutrition and hydration (MN&H).[13] The decision whether or not to use AHA should be based on the balance of benefit and harm to the patient (therapeutic ratio). If AHA can be shown to have no medical benefit for the person, and potentially to cause harm and discomfort, there is a moral duty not to initiate it or continue it.

On the other hand the 'natural' provision of food and water for oral intake is both a basic human need and a right, and no civilised person or health care institution could possibly argue for its non-provision or so-called withdrawal. It has been defined as follows: 'the provision of food and drink, to be taken voluntarily by mouth, to satisfy hunger or thirst... [This] may include physical assistance (if requested by the patient) from another person, but does not include the administration of fluids or nourishment via nasogastric tubing or an intravenous line'.[14]

The distinction between natural and artificial provision is made on the basis of what means are required to deliver the fluids and nutrients. All artificial techniques requiring intrusion on the person and medical or nursing skill for insertion and maintenance are medical treatments. In palliative care units food and drink, and assistance with eating and drinking are always available to satisfy a patient's thirst and hunger. But AHA is not routinely used when oral intake ceases, which is a normal part of the natural dying process. All treatments which are not required for comfort are stopped when a person is dying, and AHA, for example subcutaneous fluid infusion, is only used for symptomatic thirst or hunger which cannot be adequately treated by other means. Families and health care professionals are often uncomfortable with this practice. Although all therapeutic interventions should be for the benefit of the patient, the emotional needs and ethical views of the patient's family and care-givers must be acknowledged and considered. There must be recognition and fulfilment of the primary ethical duty to the patient, but the needs of those close to her or him must also be considered. The patient's decisions should determine how his or her medical treatment is to be conducted, but communication with family and friends, within the limits of respect for the patient's right to confidentiality, is almost always required. The way in which it is undertaken is a matter of skill, judgement and consultation. It should also be kept in mind that the degree of family involvement in individual patient decision-making can vary substantially between cultures.

There are two main polar approaches to decision-making at the end of life. Either the treatments or the persons to whom the treatments are applied are focused on. The two approaches are either one that would allow abatement of only certain treatments in all patients, or the other that would allow abatement of all treatments in certain patients. Somerville [15] argues against the ordinary/extraordinary distinction for deciding which treatments may morally be abated, on the grounds that it is not the treatments which tend to be so characterised but the patients to whom they are applied, and that this distinction allows subjective standards to be applied under the masquerade of objectivity. We would add the objection that it is not the moral duty of any moral, legal or medical commentator to decide *a priori* which treatments may or may not be chosen by a person or his/her substitute health care decision-maker or agent.

Objective standards

With respect to distinguishing patients, we would concur with Ramsay [16], Dyck [17], Grisez and Boyle [18] that a distinction is possible between those persons who are dying and those who are not (although we would hold some different views about treatment abatement for non-dying persons). A hard and fast objective clinical distinction as to when the dying process commences is not always possible, but *the recognition of the existence of a natural dying process is central to the ethics and practice of palliative care.* [5] The objective standards consist of clinical evidence (disease progression, vital organ failure) and overt or covert psychological evidence (from both the person who is dying and family members: anticipatory grief, emotional withdrawal, future planning which acknowledges the impending death- for example, funeral planning in the context of terminal illness). Caution should be exercised in appearing to label people as 'dying', because of the attendant dangers of depersonalisation. There is no suggestion that people who are dying have diminished rights, or that their dying days are of less value than their non-dying ones: it may be said that most people want to live until they die. Rather, their dying process should be acknowledged by all; their vulnerability increases our obligation to give care and respect, but does not lead us to give, and in fact, requires that we do not give, treatment which confers no benefit upon them.

Hydration and alimentation, including by artificial means, have become located in the category of so-called ordinary measures. Kelly [3] was the first to use the extraordinary/ordinary distinction to characterise specific treatments as either one or the other. In the orthodox interpretation of the Catholic moral tradition from which the concept is derived, as reviewed by Cronin [19] and described by McCormack [20], it is understood that it is up to individuals to decide, on the basis of proportionality, what constitutes ordinary and extraordinary treatment in their particular situation (Hepburn personal communication). A competent person determines what is ordinary or extraordinary for him/herself in the particular situation when he or she gives informed consent or informed refusal, respectively, of the medical treatment in question. If that person is no longer able to take oral nutrition or fluid, and does not wish to have these provided artificially then there the matter rests, regardless of what others have to say about the 'ordinariness' of the treatment. For an incompetent person the situation is more problematical, and there are those who would argue, as Craig appears to, that AHA cannot be abated morally or legally by anyone on behalf of an incompetent patient, particularly if the incompetence is the result of medically induced sedation. In other words she appears to propose that the provision of alimentation and hydration is a truly ordinary measure, with the means of delivery being irrelevant to the moral duty to provide them, even when a person is dying. For those who conceptualise the issues in this way, there is a clear moral and legal 'bottom-line' for the treatment that may be withheld, namely that of which provision is medically impossible or which would cause undue distress, in other words, only in the most extreme circumstances may treatment be withheld.

'Assisted feeding'

Weir [21] cites one of the most prolific and visible proponents of this position in the United States, Robert Barry OP. Barry relies on the *amicus curiae* brief of the New Jersey Catholic Conference in the Nancy Jobes case [22] and policy statements of the Committee for Pro-Life Activities of the National Conference of Bishops as evidence for his position as the correct interpretation of the tradition. Food and fluids, including AHA, should be given to all patients unless it is medically impossible to provide them. The term 'assisted feeding' is adopted to describe all provision of nutrition and hydration, and this is characterised as different from other forms of medical treatment on the grounds that death inevitably results from non-provision; less skilled expertise is required to carry it out (tubes become passive conduits); and it is 'natural'. Assisted feeding is deemed to be always morally required, and moreover it is argued that this provides an acceptable objective moral standard which can stand firm against other more subjective morally unacceptable standards and tests that might be used in treatment abatement. In short, this stance is seen as a necessary safeguard against the so-called slippery slope to morally unacceptable withholding of treatment, with the wider attendant societal effects which might ensue from AHA abatement.

A litany of suffering is listed as a consequence of starvation and dehydration, with no mention of the effects of the underlying condition. The palliative care experience has simply not been like this, and there is no basis for believing that patients receiving palliative care are dying whilst suffering from symptoms of starvation and dehydration,[13] which would be lessened or abolished by the routine provision of AHA. We agree that continual review of symptom-control profiles of patients in palliative care services is necessary-with changes in treatment where necessary, including the provision of AHA.[10]

For a potentially reversible condition, and for people with incurable conditions who are not yet dying, artificial hydration and alimentation is a medical treatment which must be offered. For incompetent persons with irreversible brain damage, the decision to cease AHA should depend on any available evidence of prior wishes of the person, and where such evidence is not available or is unclear, on their best interests, and not on a preconceived position on the obligatoriness of AHA. Nearly all the legal deliberations on the provision or withholding of AHA have been for people in this category. As Dr Craig states, the issue of AHA abatement for dying persons has not been specifically tested in the courts of the United Kingdom, and the most relevant legal deliberations are those in Airedale NHS Trust v Bland.[12] Tony Bland was not dying, but was irrefutably in a persistent vegetative state (PVS) from which no prospect of recovery was deemed possible, by all but one dissenting piece of medical evidence.[23] The judgement of the House of Lords permitted the discontinuation of AHA, which was acknowledged to be his life support, on the grounds that since it was not in his best interests (because he no longer had an interest in being alive owing to an absence of higher cognitive function) there was no duty to continue this treatment. Bland cannot be directly extrapolated to the case of dying people, as they may well be sensate until the moment of death, and often will have both an interest in being alive and the means to express that interest. Nonetheless, the deliberative process in the Bland case has been helpful to all who study decision-making at the end of life, although the court's emphasis on the act-omission distinction, with respect, may have been excessive; [24] and if the patient's best interests are identified as the main concern, the problem still remains of who determines them- it can be argued that there was an over-reliance on doctors by the court in the Bland case.

The crucial question is whether the dying person's interests are served by the provision of AHA, and this must surely be a decision based on what these measures can contribute to the person's comfort and quality of life. There are three groups of considerations to take into account in determining this. First, if these measures are requested, or are identified as necessary for comfort by the attending staff or family members, and may be effective in achieving the stated aims, then they should not be refused. It seems that there is no case law on the issue of AHA abatement for dying persons because no court has been asked specifically to consider it. This seems to indicate that in practice it has not been seen to be an issue which requires legal judgement. There is no established or accepted duty that in all cases hydration and alimentation must be maintained by whatever medical means available until death. Moreover, if AHA was not required for Bland who, unlike the dying person was not actually and actively dying of a progressive fatal condition at the time of the judgement, there is even less basis for saying that it is required for all dying persons.

Unpleasant side effects

Second, all forms of AHA carry associated unpleasant side-effects and possibly may induce premature death. The introduction of a nasogastric tube is unpleasant and its continued presence is usually a source of discomfort and irritation, and regurgitation and inhalational (overspill) pneumonia are common when patients are weak and debilitated. Venous lines can cause infective complications, and neck lines are uncomfortable and potentially hazardous to insert. Tubes and lines also become blocked or dislodged, and their replacement can be unpleasant and distressing, particularly for conscious patients with cognitive impairment. For incompetent patients in whom there is a prospect of recovery all of these problems will usually be regarded as acceptable, but the same trade-offs could not possibly apply to people who are dying.

Third, the shortening or lengthening of life can be an issue associated with the provision or non-provision of AHA. Whilst such provision or non-provision of AHA may influence the timing of an anticipated death, it is not usually possible to predict in which way, i.e. whether death would occur sooner or later than it would have done otherwise. We argue, that just as in the consideration of the issue of pain control for dying persons, the influence on timing of death should be a secondary consideration to the comfort and dignity of the dying person.

A number of legal reports and judgements have addressed treatment abatement and palliative care, and analysed the issues this raises of duties to provide care and treatment, and regarding causation of death. The non-initiation or continuation of AHA will not constitute a cause of death in the eyes of the law, if there is no duty to provide it. In such cases causation is an irrelevant consideration, because if there is no duty there can be no breach of duty which might be a cause of death of the person. From a legal point of view, in such cases the cause of death is the underlying condition which has led to the absence of oral intake, and the use of sedation for palliation of another symptom, as an essential component of care in an otherwise natural dying process, does not alter this. There is no place for emotive language about killing patients in this context.

With respect to determining when a medical practitioner has a duty to provide care, in 1982 the Canadian Law Reform Commission recommended that: 'the law should recognise that the prolonging of life is not an absolute value in itself and that therefore a physician does not act illegally when he fails to take measures to achieve this end, if these measures are useless or contrary to the patient's wishes or interests'; and: 'the law should recognise that the incapacity of a person to express his wishes is not a sufficient reason to oblige a physician to administer useless treatment for the purpose of prolonging life' and ' the law should recognise that in the case of an unconscious or incompetent patient, a physician incurs no criminal responsibility by terminating treatment that has become useless'. [25]

In other words, in each of the three sets of circumstances represented by these statements of the commission, there is no legal duty on the physician to initiate or to continue to provide useless treatment, or that which is refused by a competent person.

A court in New Zealand authorised withdrawal of ventilation from a man rendered incompetent and completely paralysed by an extreme form of Guillain-Barre syndrome. In this case, Justice Thomas throws light on what might be termed 'useless' with regard to medical care: 'Medical science and technology has advanced for a fundamental purpose: the purpose of benefiting the life and health of those who turn to medicine to be healed. It surely was never intended that it be used to prolong biological life in patients bereft of the prospect of returning to even a limited exercise of human life. Nothing in the inherent purpose of these scientific advances can require doctors to treat the dying as if they were curable. Natural death has not lost its meaning or significance. It may be deferred, but it need not be postponed indefinitely'. [26]

Gillon suggests that, where the negotiation and communication process has broken down, a mediation process should exist for situations involving differences of opinion about whether a person with a terminal illness should receive AHA. [27] This may be useful in very difficult situations, where referral to an institutional ethics committee or bioethical consultant may help. It is to be hoped that this need can usually be avoided by the sensitive and appropriate raising of the issues addressed in this paper. Due regard is, however, required for the cultural and ethnic dimensions involved. Families who feel that they are neglecting their role and duty in the provision of nourishment will not appreciate having a discussion about the ethical or legal issues raised in relation to treatment abatement. They are, however, much more likely to agree to a care plan which is gently worked out with them, where all parties agree on their common values concerning the comfort, value and integrity of the person who is dying, and the absence of anyone's responsibility for that dying.

In conclusion, we believe that the approach which we have described here is the dominant one in modern palliative care practice, and is accepted in the mainstream of contemporary ethical discourse. We agree with Beauchamp and Childress who see: '…no reason to believe that medically administered nutrition and hydration is always an essential part of palliative care or that it necessarily constitutes, on balance, a beneficial medical treatment'. [13]

Acknowledgements

Michael Ashby was supported by the Special Purposes Fund of the Royal Adelaide Hospital. Thanks to the director (Professor Margaret Somerville) and staff of the Centre for Medicine, Ethics and Law, McGill University, Montreal, Quebec, Canada and to Dr Liz Hepburn IBVM, Director of the Provincial Bioethics Centre for the Dioceses of Queensland, for their assistance in writing this paper.

Michael Ashby, MBBS, MRCP (UK), FRCR, FRACP, MRACMA, is Professor of Palliative Care, Monash University, based at Monash Medical Centre, Clayton, Victoria 3168. Brian Stoffell, BA, PhD, is Director, Medical Ethics Unit, Flinders Medical Centre and Flinders University of South Australia.

References

1. Craig GM. On withholding nutrition and hydration in the terminally ill: has palliative medicine gone too far? *Journal of Medical Ethics* 1994; **20**: 139-143.

2. Ashby MA, Stoffell B. Therapeutic ration and defined phases: proposal of ethical framework for palliative care. *British Medical Journal* 1991; **302:** 1322-1324.

3. Kelly G. *Medico-moral problems*. St Louis: the Catholic Hospital Association of US and Canada, 1954; 6-15.

4. *Cancer pain relief and palliative care*. Technical Report Series 804. Geneva: World Health Organisation, 1990.

5. Ashby MA, Brooksbank MA, Stoffell B. Natural death and the ethics of palliative care. [In preparation].

6. Hunt R. Palliative care- the rhetoric-reality gap. In: Kuhse H, ed. *Willing to listen, wanting to die*. Melbourne: Penguin Australia, 1994.

7. Wilkes E. On withholding nutrition and hydration in the terminally ill: has palliative medicine gone too far? A commentary. *Journal of Medical Ethics* 1994; **20**: 144-145.

8. Haines IE, Zalcberg J, Buchanan JD. Not-for-resuscitation-orders in cancer patients- principles of decision making. *Medical Journal of Australia* 1990; **153**: 225-229.

9. Fainsinger R, Bruera E. The management of dehydration in terminally ill patients. *Journal of Palliative Care* 1994; **10**: 55-59.

10. Bruera E, Legris MA, Kuehn N, Miller MJ. Hypodermoclysis for the administration of fluids and narcotic analgesics in patients with advanced cancer. *Journal of Pain and Symptom Management* 1990; **5**: 218-220.

11. Callahan D. *The troubled dream of life*: *living with mortality*. New York: Simon Shuster, 1993.

12. Airedale NHS Trust v Bland. {1993} 1 ALL ER 821-896.

13. Beauchamp TL, and Childress JF. Principles of biomedical ethics. New York: Oxford University Press, 1994.

14. Ashby M. Law reform on death- over but not out. *Australian Health Law Bulletin* 1994; **2**: 81-85.

15. Somerville M. Advice to the Minister of Health of South Australia on the Consent to Medical Treatment and Palliative Care Bill, Dec 1992 {unpublished}

16. Ramsay P. Prolonged dying: not medically indicated. *Hastings Center Report* 1976; **6**: 14-17.

17. Dyck A. Ethical aspects of caring for the dying incompetent. *Journal of the American Geriatric Society* 1984; **32**: 661-664.

18. Grisez G, Boyle JM. *Life and death with liberty and justice*. Notre Dame, Indiana: University of Notre Dame Press, 1979.
19. Cronin DA. Conserving human life. Doctorial dissertation [1958] republished in Cronin DA. *Conserving human life*. Boston, Ma: The Pope John Center, 1989.
20. McCormack R. The quality of life, the sanctity of life. *Hastings Center Report* 1978; **1**: 30-36.
21. Weir RF. *Abating treatment with critically ill patients*. New York: Oxford, 1989.
22. In re Jobes, 108 NJ. 394, 529 A. 2d 434 (1987)
23. Andrews K. Patients in the persistent vegetative state: problems in their long term management. *British Medical Journal* 1993; **306**: 1600-1602.
24. Collins D. *Prescribing limits to life long treatment*. AIC Medical Conference. Auckland 1994 Apr 19-20.
25. Law Reform Commission of Canada. *Protection of life: euthanasia, aiding suicide and cessation of treatment*. Working paper 28. Ottawa, 1982.
26. Auckland AHA v A-G. [1993] 1 NZLR 235.
27. Gillon R. Palliative care ethics: non-provision of artificial nutrition and hydration to terminally ill sedated patients. *Journal of Medical Ethics* 1994; **20**: 131-132.

The debate continued in the columns of the Journal of Medical Ethics with another paper by Craig. This started as a letter drafted in reply to a point made by Ashby and Stoffell, but grew into a review of the published debate during the years 1994-1996. Shortly before publication the judgement in a test case in Scotland came through, bringing Scottish case law in line with that in England and Wales as determined by the case of Airedale NHS Trust v Bland. And so the debate continued as follows....

Chapter 5

The Debate Continues

On withholding artificial hydration and nutrition from terminally ill sedated patients. The debate continues

Gillian M Craig *retired Consultant Geriatrician, Northampton*
Journal of Medical Ethics 1996; 22: 147-153.

Abstract

The author reviews and continues the debate initiated by her recent paper in this journal.[1] The paper was critical of certain aspects of palliative medicine, and caused Ashby and Stoffell to modify the framework they proposed in 1991.[2] It now takes account of the need for artificial hydration to satisfy thirst, or other symptoms due to lack of fluid intake in the terminally ill [7] There is also a more positive attitude to the emotional needs and ethical views of the patient's family and care-givers.

However, clinical concerns about the general reluctance to use artificial hydration in terminal care remain, and doubts persist about the ethical and legal arguments used by some palliative medicine specialists and others, to justify their approach. Published contributions to the debate to date, in professional journals are reviewed. Key statements relating to the care of sedated terminally ill patients are discussed, and where necessary criticised.

Introduction

I welcome the discussion that has been generated by my paper in this journal, on the subject of withholding nutrition and hydration in the terminally ill.' I criticised a framework for palliative care advocated by Ashby and Stoffell.[2] My central theme was the issue of the need for artificial hydration when a patient is rendered incapable of swallowing by sedation. I argued that to withhold hydration is dangerous medically, ethically and legally. and can be disturbing for relatives.

At the time of writing I am aware of four papers and two letters that have been published in reply in this journal [3-8] and two papers elsewhere.[9,10] Gillon touched on legal aspects and raised the question of the need for formal mediation procedures.[3] Wilkes, in a gentle and broadly-based commentary, shared some of my anxieties,[4] Ashby and Stoffell continued the debate in a wide-ranging response [7] and others focused on clinical aspects.[8,10] The issues raised have been considered by the ethics committee of the Association for Palliative Medicine in the United Kingdom, by the board of the Cancer Relief Macmillan Fund, and by senior people in many walks of life. This paper summarises and extends the debate as it has developed in professional journals.

The subject under discussion straddles the boundaries of medicine, ethics and law, and strays into other academic areas too. The debate could easily get out of hand. In replying to papers that have appeared to date, I will not engage in detailed discussion of concepts such as care, needs, proportionality of medical interventions and processes of communication, although the discussion that follows touches on these issues in several places. To shift the focus of the argument into these areas, as proposed by Ashby and Stoffell,[7] could be detrimental to progress. There are matters arising which need to be clarified before the agenda moves on. It is important to continue the debate on a level that will be of practical assistance to medical practitioners and possibly lawyers, who may be embroiled in the management of these difficult cases.

Clinical aspects

Need for artificial hydration in some circumstances is acknowledged

I am glad to say that Ashby and Stoffell have amended their framework for palliative care to take account of some of my criticisms. They now say, with some preamble, that "artificial hydration may be required in the terminal phase to satisfy thirst, or other symptoms due to lack of fluid intake", and admit that "the emotional needs and ethical views of the patient's family and care-givers must be acknowledged and considered". They add that "if artificial hydration and nutrition are identified as necessary for comfort by attending staff or family members, and may be effective in achieving the stated aims, then they should not be refused.[7]

Dunlop et al agree that there are rare occasions when it is justifiable to give subcutaneous fluids for the sake of the family, but do not recommend the routine use of intravenous or subcutaneous fluids. They distinguish between sedation used in terminal delirium, and sedation used in patients who are not actually dying. They imply that in the latter situation problems with hydration rarely occur and so their discussion stops short of the ethical dilemma at issue.[8]

Dunphy et al in a brave and balanced discussion of the whole issue of rehydration in palliative or terminal care, stress the need to make "genuine and unprejudged assessments of the relevance of dehydration to each individual's clinical presentation, and above all to be responsive to the wishes of the family." [10]

Risks of artificial hydration are exaggerated

Ashby and Stoffell exaggerate the risks of artificial hydration quite considerably.[7] Dunlop et al comment that no studies to their knowledge have demonstrated any adverse effects from fluid therapy, but advise caution if the serum albumin is low.[8] Artificial hydration could be harmful in patients with cerebral oedema,[5] cardiac failure, or any condition where symptoms are related to fluid overload. There will also be situations where fluid restriction is helpful, for example in patients with inappropriate secretion of anti-diuretic hormone - a condition that is found in some patients with cancer. All medical intervention must be used with clinical discretion. Some patients may benefit initially from a reduction in fluid intake, or cessation of artificial hydration and alimentation (AHA), but no one can survive indefinitely without sustenance.

Risk of misdiagnosis and undertreatment

Ashby and Stoffell fail to understand the basis for my general concern. They take a comment about the need to buy time for assessment by energetic rehydration as a cue to launch into a tirade about technological brinkmanship. Yet they admit that when accepting patients for palliative care they have to "insist on fuller clinical information than some referring doctors think is really necessary for palliative care". The inference to be drawn is that patients are being labelled as terminal on inadequate grounds which, to coin a phrase used by Ashby and Stoffell, is my point entirely. The case reports I gave to illustrate this point were dismissed as "hard cases which can be mobilised to undermine any approach". Actually they were hard cases that could represent the tip of an iceberg. Who knows how many patients die at home, or in hospital labelled as terminal, misdiagnosed and undertreated? As Wilkes observed, dehydration occurs far too frequently, far removed from the territory of palliative care.[4]

Artificial nutrition

Dunlop *et al* rightly consider hydration and nutrition as separate issues.[8] My main concerns relate to hydration, as the need for long term nutritional support with all its potential difficulties will rarely arise in terminal care. Although the administration of conventional dextrose solutions via a peripheral vein does not constitute full nutritional support,[8] it does provide some useful calories in the short term, and is often given on medical and surgical wards for one or two weeks, to tide over patients who cannot eat. Dextrose solutions should not be given subcutaneously.

The question of thirst

Ashby and Stoffell claim that I allege that sedation is used to mask the effects of dehydration or starvation.[7] I did not say this, although it may well be so in some cases. On the question of thirst in general there is a hint of irritation and dismissal in their response to my comments, and they fail to appreciate that it is the relatives' concern about suffering that I describe. It is no good brusquely referring people to the literature. Jo Blogs is not aware of the literature, all he sees is someone apparently dying of thirst or starving to death. That is the public perception of the situation, and in some cases they could be right. Moreover the literature is not uniformly reassuring on this point.

McCann and co-workers found thirst and/or a dry mouth to be a major symptom in 66% of 32 patients initially, with hunger being less of a problem, despite severe protein-calorie malnutrition.[11] Thirst tended to decrease as death approached, despite probable dehydration. Anorexia may have been due to fasting, underlying disease or narcotic administration.[11] Dunlop *et al* comment that most terminally ill cancer patients reach a point during their general decline when they first stop eating, and subsequently stop drinking.[8] They make the interesting suggestion that the normal homeostatic mechanisms controlling fluid intake and fluid balance may be altered in the dying process. All the evidence in support of this suggestion needs to be carefully and impartially reviewed, but the letter by Waller to which they refer is open to criticism.[6]

Much remains to be discovered about the pathophysiological sequence of events, as some changes may prove to be reversible. Does severe dehydration, for example, suppress thirst in cancer patients, as it does in the healthy elderly?* If so the result would be an escalating spiral of decline. Is it not time that someone studied the beneficial effects of rehydration in terminal care?

Clearly if patients have stopped drinking because of an irreversible decline it is one thing, but if they are suddenly rendered incapable of eating or drinking by sedation it is another. It is the latter situation that creates ethical problems.

The need to keep intervention simple

I am not advocating artificial hydration and nutrition in all dying patients irrespective of the circumstances, nor did I propose, as Ashby and Stoffell try to imply, "that provision of alimentation and hydration is a truly ordinary measure, with the means of delivery being irrelevant... even when a person is dying."[7] I argued that a drip or subcutaneous infusion is a simple, ordinary and effective procedure, that rarely causes the patient discomfort or distress, and should be used more readily in a hospice setting.[1] I agree that to advocate measures such as gastrostomy or total parenteral nutrition when death is imminent and unavoidable, would be inappropriate. However, as others comment: "It may be that the issue we need to address is our assessment of likely benefit, rather than attempting to quantify medical intrusion."[10]

Ashby and Stoffell complain that excessive reliance on technology can have unfortunate consequences for medical practice. One consequence is the introduction of advance directives, or living wills, by those who wish to protect themselves from the worst excesses of technology, or who, conversely, wish to be treated. Difficulties in medicine may now arise, not only for doctors who wish to discontinue treatment in the dying,[7] but also for those who wish to treat their patients and return them from imminent death to life. Not all of us share the view of the fictional doctor who said "I have every confidence that the law is not such an ass that it will force me to watch a patient of mine die unnecessarily."[12] None of these problems would have arisen, had doctors proved better at walking the tight-rope between over-treatment and under-treatment. Excessive swings in either direction need to be curbed, and a balanced approach achieved.

The legal question

Legal matters are covered in some detail by Ashby and Stoffell, assisted by Professor M Somerville and the staff of the Centre for Medicine, Ethics and Law of McGill University, and by a bioethicist from Queensland.[7] In wide-ranging discussion, scattered throughout their response they refer to papers on the distinction between natural and artificial provision of fluid and nourishment and conclude that the latter constitutes medical treatment. This remains somewhat contentious. On the subject of the limits to a medical practitioner's duty to care, they quote recommendations made by the Canadian Law Commission in 1982. Reference to the established law as it applies in the

[*Note. This point was clarified later - see page 70]

United Kingdom would have been more relevant. They quote the comments of a judge in New Zealand to illustrate what might be termed "useless" with regard to medical care, but, with respect, the situation of a man rendered incompetent and paralysed by an extreme form of Guillain-Barré syndrome does not equate with the clinical situation under discussion. All in all, this international sledge-hammer approach does not crack the kernel of the problem, which is whether sedation without hydration or nutrition in terminal care is legal in the UK. Indeed it makes focused debate rather more difficult. I have, however, selected some key issues for discussion. Others would no doubt choose a different path through the legal and ethical maze.

1. The futility argument

It is often said that a doctor has no duty to continue a treatment that is useless and of no benefit to the patient - but as others have observed, futility is not always the ethical trump card that some would like it to be.[13] Ashby and Stoffell argue that "It is possibly true that sedation may hasten the actual time at which relatively imminent death will occur. But it is not deemed necessary to hydrate sedated patients during the dying process when they are unable to maintain oral intake, as it makes no sense to attempt to treat a transiently reversible component of their overall dying process".

This is not a terribly satisfactory response to the dilemma presented. From a legal standpoint the provision of hydration may be crucial, particularly since Ashby and Stoffell stress elsewhere in their paper that "from a legal point of view ... the cause of death is the underlying condition which has led to the absence of oral intake" ... (i.e. in some cases sedation) ... and that "non-provision of artificial hydration can shorten life."[7]

We need to consider the case of a patient who is not dying, or in whom death is not relatively imminent. Such a patient may need sedation, perhaps for intractable pain, and could become fatally dehydrated as a consequence. Clearly some people would consider hydration of such a patient futile, and so it may be if the end point sought is restoration of the patient to health. Or consider the case of a stroke patient, confused and perhaps aphasic, whose prospects of recovery are judged to be poor, and who may have swallowing difficulties in addition. Many such patients get dehydrated even without sedation, and some physicians take an inactive approach to management.

Is there any good reason why treatment decisions made about such patients should be any less rigorous than those required for incompetent patients? In the latter case "as long as the patient is alive, the legal justification for providing treatment is the principle of necessity."[14] Treatment is "necessary" provided that it is in the "best interests" of patients, and this occurs "if, but only if, it is carried out either to save their lives, or to ensure improvement, or prevent deterioration in their physical or mental health."[15]

Sometimes in the case of terminally ill or physically disabled patients, it is tacitly assumed that it is in their best interests that they should die. Yet in cases of doubt, especially where survival outcome or prognosis is uncertain, the balance should be weighted in favour of prolonging life.

Even when death is inevitable, the simple and safe measure of a subcutaneous infusion may not be futile. It may be of some help to the patient, and may comfort the relatives, calm their fears, and reduce the incidence of pathological grief and post-traumatic stress reactions. It may also reassure all concerned that the patient died of his or her disease, rather than the treatment. Thus it could avert the need for lengthy, costly and distressing inquiries after death.

2. Case studies in English, Irish and Scottish law

There is still no case law on the issue of abatement of artificial hydration and alimentation in the dying, and the most relevant legal deliberations relate to the case of Airedale Trust v Bland in England,[16] the Irish Supreme Court case in the Republic of Ireland,' [17][18] and the case of Mrs Johnstone of Lanarkshire, which has clarified the law regarding patients with a persistent vegetative state (PVS) in Scotland.' [19]

The Bland case ruling applied strictly, and only, to the situation in that case [16,20] and should not be extrapolated to other clinical situations.[1] However, Ashby and Stoffell have done just that, saying "...if AHA was not required for Bland, who unlike the dying person was not actually or actively dying of a progressive fatal condition at the time of the judgement, there is even less basis for saying that it is required for all dying persons." [7] This is a very rash statement. Firstly no one is saying that AHA is required for all dying persons. Secondly some patients who require sedation in palliative care are not actually dying, nor are they necessarily unconscious. Thirdly the statement demonstrates an alarming lack of appreciation of the exceedingly careful ethical and legal deliberations that led to the decision in the Bland case. If society takes a decision about one patient with PVS so seriously, surely equally serious thought should be given to matters of hydration and nutrition in sedated patients with incurable disease. The shorter time scale in the dying does not eliminate the legal and ethical dilemmas. Fourthly the statement overlooks the major differences in mental state and underlying pathology between a terminally ill patient who is sedated, and a patient with PVS.

The Irish Supreme Court case

This concerned a 45-year-old woman in a near PVS, who retained some ability to recognise people, but could not move or communicate, following brain damage sustained in a minor operation 23 years earlier. The court ruled in May 1995 that she could be allowed to die by withdrawal of nourishment. The chief justice took the view that the true cause of the woman's death would be the injuries she sustained in 1973, and not withdrawal of nourishment.[17] Mr Justice Lynch said that what he had to decide was not the morality of the course that the family sought to follow, but the lawfulness of it.[18]

The Irish Medical Council, in a statement issued in August 1995,[21] saw no need to alter its ethical guidelines, so leaving any doctor who assisted in withdrawing AHA open to disciplinary action. The council emphasised certain paragraphs which are of relevance to the present discussion.

- Doctors must do their best to preserve life and promote the health of the sick person.
- Medical care must not be used as a tool of the state to be granted or withheld or altered in character under political pressure.
- Where death is imminent, it is the doctor's responsibility to take care that a patient dies with dignity and with as little suffering as possible. Euthanasia, which involves deliberately causing the death of a patient, is professional misconduct and is illegal in Ireland.
- They also quoted articles two and four of Principles of Medical Ethics in Europe [21]:
- Article 2: In the course of his medical practice a doctor undertakes to give priority to the medical interests of the patient. The doctor may use his professional knowledge only to improve or maintain the health of those who place their trust in him; in no circumstances may he act to their detriment.
- Article 4: ... The doctor must not substitute his own definition of the quality of life for that of his patient.

Finally the Irish Medical Council added their view that "access to nutrition and hydration is one of the basic needs of human beings. This remains so even when, from time to time, this need can only be fulfilled by means of long-established methods such as naso-gastric and gastrostomy tube feeding." [21]

The Scottish Court of Session case. Law Hospital Trust v Johnstone

The final judgment in the case of Mrs Janet Johnstone, who has had PVS for four years following a drug overdose, was given recently. According to reports in *The Guardian*,[19] Lord Cameron of Lochbroom, after hearing evidence, passed the case on to the Inner House of the Court of Session for legal guidance. Five senior judges headed by Lord President Hope, declared that Lord Cameron would, if he chose, be entitled to grant requests that artificial feeding be abandoned. However, they warned that they had had no right to grant Mrs Johnstone's doctors immunity from prosecution for murder. Scotland's senior law officer, the Lord Advocate, Lord Mackay of Drumadoon later stated that he would not "authorise the prosecution of a qualified medical practitioner (or any person acting on the instructions of such a practitioner) who, acting in good faith and with the authority of the Court of Session, withdraws or otherwise causes to be discontinued life-sustaining treatment or other medical treatment from a patient in a persistent, or permanent vegetative state, with the result that the patient dies". Permission to cease AHA was finally granted by Lord Cameron.' [19] Immunity from prosecution cannot automatically be extended to treatment-limiting decisions in the dying, or the disabled. Society is now, rather painfully, through the courts, deciding where the line should be drawn.

It cannot be said that there is universal agreement that AHA can be regarded as medical treatment that can be stopped if deemed to be futile. Grave doubts remain, as evidenced by the Irish Medical Council's statement, Lord Mustill's unease concerning the Bland case,[16] the views of the House of Lord's Select

Committee on Medical Ethics,[22] and comments made by the Hon Mr Justice Ognall when discussing the hypothetical case of a patient whose severe pain could only be controlled by general anaesthesia.[23] He drew attention to subtleties of distinction between switching off a life support system, as in the Bland case, and the withdrawal of nutrition and hydration in the latter situation.[23] The House of Lords Select Committee were unable to reach a decision about whether nutrition and hydration, even when given by invasive methods, may ever be regarded as treatment, which in certain circumstances it may be inappropriate to initiate or continue.[22]

3. The principle of double effect

The medical profession, supported by the legal profession, tend to shelter behind the principle of double effect. Ashby and Stoffell are no exception, arguing that "the influence on timing of death should be of secondary consideration to the comfort and dignity of the dying person".[7]

The principle of double effect was used by the judge in the case of R v Adams in 1957. It was alleged that Dr Adams had killed a patient affected by a stroke, by giving large doses of heroin and morphine. He was acquitted, the judge saying: "If the first purpose of medicine, the restoration of health can no longer be achieved, there is still much for the doctor to do, and he is entitled to do all that is proper and necessary to relieve pain and suffering, even if the measures he takes may incidentally shorten life." [21] Forty years on standards of medicine have changed. If all that is proper and necessary is done, there should rarely be any need for life to be shortened.

Anglican and Catholic Bishops have recently reaffirmed their support for the principle of double effect, noting that "There is a proper and fundamental ethical distinction ... between that which is intended and that which is foreseen but unintended." [25]

I have argued elsewhere that the principle of double effect is open to abuse, and could be quoted in the defence of medical practitioners whose standards of care and intentions are open to question. Where the side-effects of a treatment, such as sedation, are predictable, potentially lethal, and easily overcome by simple measures, failure to use such measures could be regarded as negligent.[9] Some witnesses to the House of Lords Select Committee also expressed concern and suggested that the double effect of some therapeutic drugs, when given in large doses, was being used as a cloak for euthanasia. The committee, however, expressed confidence in the medical profession, and in the ability of a jury to evaluate a doctor's intention.[26] The profession must prove worthy of such public trust.

4. The euthanasia question

Notwithstanding the objections raised by Ashby and Stoffell who say "there is no place for emotive language about killing patients in this context," [7] a consideration of this matter is not out of place in this debate. I posed the questions: "Are you, by withholding fluid and nourishment, withholding the means of sustaining life? In short are you killing the patient?"

Gillon refers to moral distinctions between killing, and letting die.[3] The Hon Mr Justice Ognall points out that "the distinction between deliberate acts intended to kill ... and letting die ... is not free from difficulties. Is a doctor who allows a terminally ill patient to die guilty of murder? Our law says no, but, providing his intention in omitting to act is to hasten the patient's death, what is the distinction in that circumstance between an act on the one hand, and an omission on the other?"[23]

The current legal position regarding euthanasia in Scotland, England and Wales involves two elements: "a) a guilty act and b) the necessary intent. In general an omission to prevent death is not a guilty act, and cannot give rise to a conviction for murder. But where the accused was under a duty to the deceased, for example as his parent, nurse or doctor, to carry out the act which he omitted to do, such omission could be sufficient for the crime of either murder or culpable homicide, depending on the intention of the accused."[22]

Thus the question of whether the practice of sedation without hydration or nourishment in terminal care is legal, can only be decided by careful consideration of all the facts in an individual case.

Other matters

Who should decide?

Ashby and Stoffell end a rather tortuous paragraph on decision-making at the end of life, with the objection that "It is not the duty of any moral, legal or medical commentator to decide a *priori,* which treatment may or may not be chosen by a person or his/her substitute health care decision-maker or agent."[7]

This sweeping statement takes us into the mine-field of patient autonomy, and to a consideration of the adverse effects that this can have on a physician's authority, and on the whole equilibrium of the health care team. The tensions created account for many of the difficulties that dissenting relatives or attendant staff may experience. Such tension will be greatest where life and death decisions are involved. It can also be sensed when a dissenting colleague questions "received wisdom" in the journals! For a philosophical overview on autonomy, see Norden.[12] The nurse/physician authority relationship is explored by May.[28]

From a purely practical point of view there may be no problem if the patient is able to make his or her views about treatment known. Substitute healthcare decision-makers, however, have no legal standing in the UK at present. Problems arise when treatment-limiting decisions must be made for an incompetent patient. The House of Lords Select Committee on Medical Ethics advised that in this situation "decisions should be made by all those involved in his or her care, including the whole health care team, and the family or other people closest to the patient. Their guiding principle should be that a treatment may be judged inappropriate if it will add nothing to the patient's well being as a person."[22] The principle of necessity referred to above is also pertinent.

I drew attention to the problems that can arise when relatives or members of the health care team request intervention such as hydration, in terminally ill patients.[1] Ashby and Stoffell believe that the sensitivities and consultative processes required to handle such a situation are already embodied in contemporary palliative care practice. I would say that there is much room for improvement and no cause for complacency. Their penultimate paragraph hints at persuasion of the family to accept treatment abatement.[7] One cannot help feeling that anyone who requested active intervention, for any reason, would need to be exceedingly persuasive, determined and articulate to achieve it. The more gentle, flexible and unqualified approach to the family adopted by Dunlop *et al* is preferable.[8]

The need for formal mediation procedures

Gillon drew attention to the need for some formal mediation procedure in British hospitals and hospices,[3] but little progress has been made on this point. However, there are encouraging signs, in the form of a thoughtful paper on the subject of clinical ethics committees, from the Institute of Epidemiology and Health Services Research in Leeds.[29]

Some thoughts on care and compassion

A physician can work for a lifetime with care and compassion without pausing to analyse these sentiments, or read books on the subject. There is an approach to ethics based on care, which some view as hopelessly vague.[30] Some Buddhist and Christian views have been discussed in this journal recently, and are relevant to this debate.[25] The word care itself, is in danger of being devalued, since those who campaign for the right to die in Oregon, USA, see their action as a campaign for compassionate care. No doubt they are motivated by sadness and pity in response to pain and disability, but compassion need not kill. "It is unsafe to encourage or even to allow compassion to see death as its only or prime instrument."[31]

There is correct compassion and correct care. Anglican and Catholic Bishops refer to the …"Special care and protection" … that the vulnerable deserve … "which provides a fundamental test as to what constitutes a civilised society."[25] "Good medicine involves compassion, but it must be correct compassion leading to constructive action."[32] Doctors should care for the patient supportively and wisely, care for the relatives sensitively, and care for the carers.

Finally there is the legal view of a doctor's duty to care, some aspects of which have been mentioned already.[1,7,27] As the Irish Supreme Court case showed, legal and medical opinions in this area do not always agree. There is clearly a need for doctors, lawyers and ethicists to find more common ground, but standards must not be compromised for political or economic reasons. In the context of the care of the dying it is essential that the law of double effect is honoured, and not abused.[9]

Some thoughts on needs

This debate has highlighted the needs of the terminally ill patient for comfort and supportive care, the needs of the relatives, and the need for formal mediation procedures. Doctors and nurses also need to recognise that their own values, attitudes to disability, training and experience will influence their decision-making. Some may consider that there are fates worse than death, but as the Leicester hospice team report, "even a terminally ill patient with incurable malignancy may find life worthwhile and precious." [33] There is a need for research into the value of maintaining hydration, so that treatment can be evidence-based. At present, as Dunphy *et al* point out, it may be that a patient's place of care, whether hospital, hospice or home, is the main factor that determines whether he or she is rehydrated or not.[10] The view that access to nutrition and hydration is a basic human need, irrespective of the means by which it is delivered [21] is profoundly important. Access to nutrition and hydration determines whether a person lives or dies, whether on a hospital ward, or during famine or war. Decisions about AHA give society, through doctors, considerable power over life and death. Such power must be used with the utmost responsibility.

Summary

This debate has proved valuable. On clinical aspects the responses to date have shown a refreshing willingness by palliative medicine specialists to examine and question their clinical practice.[10] Some have modified certain aspects of their practice but have defended others vigorously.[7] There is some measure of agreement that careful assessment of individual patients is essential, and that some will benefit from rehydration.[10, 6] Hydration can be maintained quite simply using the subcutaneous route in the patient's home if need be.[34]

Legal and ethical discussion has highlighted areas of great difficulty. Consideration of cases such as the Bland case, though necessary, has tended to deflect attention away from the central issue of the use of sedation without hydration in terminal care. However, discussion has been greatly helped by the deliberations of the House of Lord's Select Committee on Medical Ethics.[22] They made it clear that it should be unnecessary to consider the withdrawal of nutrition or hydration except in circumstances where its administration is in itself a burden to the patient. Careful consideration of the benefit/burden equation in individual patients is of central importance to patient management.

We all want the dying to depart in peace, in comfort and with dignity. We should all try to ensure that their relatives have peace of mind too. Of course we are not required to "treat the dying as if they were curable" [35] — but we are required to support life wisely, until it comes to a natural end. That is the whole purpose of this debate.

References and notes

1   Craig GM. On withholding nutrition and hydration in the terminally ill: has palliative medicine gone too far? *Journal of Medical Ethics* 1994; **20**: 139-43.

2   Ashby M, Stoffel B. Therapeutic ratio and defined phases: proposal of ethical framework for palliative care. *British Medical Journal* 1991; **302**: 1322-4.

3   Gillon R [editorial]. Palliative care ethics: non-provision of artificial nutrition and hydration to terminally ill sedated patients. *Journal of Medical Ethics* 1994; **20:** 131-2, 187.

4   Wilkes E. On withholding nutrition and hydration in the terminally ill: has palliative medicine gone too far? A commentary. *Journal of Medical Ethics* 1994; **20:**144-5.

5   Stone P, Phillips C [letter]. Nutrition, dehydration and the terminally ill. *Journal of Medical Ethics* 1995; **21:**55.

6   Craig G. M [letter]. Nutrition, dehydration and the terminally ill. *Journal of Medical Ethics* 1995; **21**: 184-5.

7   Ashby M, Stoffell B. Artificial hydration and alimentation at the end of life: a reply so Craig. *Journal of Medical Ethics* 1995; **21**: 135-40.

8   Dunlop R, EllershawJE, Baines MJ, Sykes N, Saunders C. On withholding nutrition and hydration in the terminally ill: has palliative medicine gone too far? A reply. *Journal of Medical Ethics.* 1995; **21**: 141-3.

9   Craig G. M. Is sedation without hydration or nourishment in terminal care lawful? *Medico-legal Journal* 1994; **62**: 198-201.

10 Dunphy K, Finly I, Rathbone G, Gilbert J, Hick F. Rehydration in palliative and terminal care: if not — why not? *Palliative Medicine* 1995; **9**: 221-8.

11 McCann R M, Hall W J, Groth-Juncker A. Comfort care for terminally ill patients. The appropriate use of nutrition and hydration. *Journal of the American Medical Association.* 1994; **272**: 1263-6.

12 Norden M. Medicine and literature: *Whose Life Is It Anyway?* A study in respect for autonomy. *Journal of Medical Ethics* 1995; **21**: 179-83.

13 Weijer C, Elliott C. Pulling the plug on futility. *British Medical Journal* 1995; **310**: 683-4.

14 Jones M A. The legal background. *British Medical Journal* 1995; **310**: 717.

15 F v West Berkshire Health Authority. 1989.2 All ER 545,551. See ref. 14.

16 House of Lords. Law Report. Withdrawal of medical treatment from hopeless case not unlawful. *The Times* 1993 Feb 5: 8.

17 Murdoch A news report *British Medical Journal* 1995; **311**: 405.

18 Sharrock D. Irish court rules that woman in coma for years be allowed to die. *The Guardian* 1995 May 6: 2 (col 2).

19 Clouston E, Dyer C. Life or death decision goes to Lord Advocate. *The Guardian* 1996 Mar 23: 6 (cola 1-6), and Dyer C. Legal threat lifted from coma cases. *The Guardian* 1996 Apt 12: 7 (cols 1-3) and Dyer C. Judge rules doctors can let coma woman die. *The Guardian* 1996 April 25: 7 (cols 1-2).

20 McLean S. Making advance medical decisions. *Journal of the Medical and Dental Defence Unions* 1995; **34**:28-9.
21 Irish Medical Council Statement. 1995 Aug 4. Medical Council, Portobello Court, Lower Rathmines Road, Dublin 6. Articles 2 and 4 are translated from *Principes d'Ethique Medicale Européenne.* Report of the Conference International des Ordres et des Organismes d'Attributions Similaires, Paris, 1987. Published by Le Conseil Nationale de l'Ordre des Médécins, 60 Boulevard de Latour-Maubourg Paris 75007, France.
22 House of Lords Select Committee. *Report on medical ethics.* London: HMSO, 1994: para 251-257.
23 Ognall H. A right to die? Some medico-legal reflection. *Medico-legal Journal* 1994; **4**:165-179.
24 Young A. In the patient's interests. Law and professional conduct. In: Hunt G. ed. *Ethical issues in nursing.* London: Routledge, 1994:165.
25 Keown D, Keown J. Killing, karma and caring: euthanasia in Buddhism and Christianity. *Journal of Medical Ethics* 1995; **21**: 265-9.
26 See reference 22: paras 242 and 243 and reference 23: 172-3.
27 Euthanasia. Section 7.3. *Report of the Board of Social Responsibility of the Church of Scotland.* 1994: para 4.1.
28 May T. The basis and limits of physician authority: a *reply to critics.* *Journal of Medical Ethics* 1995; **21**: 170-3.
29 Thoruton JG, Lilford RJ. Clinical ethics committees. *British Medical Journal* 1995; **311**: 667-9.
30 Allmark P. Can there be an ethics of care? *Journal of Medical Ethics* 1995; **21**: 19-24.
31 See reference 27: para 5.8.
32 Grimley Evans J. Technology and the quality of life of the elderly. The Churches' Council on Health and Healing Conference on *The Moral and Spiritual Implications of Medical Technology* London, 1995 Nov
33 Meystre CJN, Alunedzai 5, Burley NMJ [letter]. Terminally ill patients may want to live. *British Medical Journal* 1994; **309**: 409.
34 McQuillan R, Finlay I. Dehydration in dying patients. *Palliative Medicine* 1995; **9**: 341-2.
35 See reference 7 p139.

Thirst and hydration in palliative care.

Craig G.M.
Letter published in the Journal of Medical Ethics 1996; 22 (6) :361.
© BMJ Publishing Group. Reprinted with permission.

SIR,
I write to correct an error in my recent paper in your journal,[1] and to clarify and expand a point relating to the physiology of thirst.

Physiology of thirst

The physiology of thirst is extremely complex, and my knowledge of it rather rusty. In touching on it I have made a statement that is misleading. On page 148 of my paper in the section on "The question of thirst" I wrote: "Does severe dehydration suppress thirst in cancer patients as it does in the healthy elderly?" In fact is probably not dehydration that suppresses thirst in the elderly, but suppression of thirst that predisposes to dehydration.[2] Phillips et al showed reduced thirst during fluid deprivation in seven healthy elderly men, compared with seven healthy young men.[2] The reason for this was not clear but the authors postulated diminished baroreceptor and volume receptor mediated thirst since levels of the peptide hormone vasopressin, which is linked with osmoreceptors [3] were not reduced. However, certain odd features in the study suggested that cognitive factors were involved, since thirst levels that were suppressed during fluid deprivation, rose during a subsequent "sham" intravenous infusion. Therefore the knowledge that one cannot have access to fluids, may lead to thirst suppression. The important point however is that the combination of dehydration and thirst suppression, whatever the mechanism, is potentially lethal, and could indeed lead to "an escalating spiral of decline."

In the context of a possible reduction in thirst perception in the dying' it is of interest that loss of osmotic thirst has been reported in patients with multiple system atrophy.[3] It is also of interest that opiates play a part in the control of vasopressin secretion,[4] as may prostaglandins [5] Whether this alters thirst perception I do not know, but clearly morphine and other pain-killers used in palliative care could influence fluid-balance control in unpredictable ways.

References

1. Craig G. M. On withholding artificial hydration and nutrition from terminally ill sedated patients. The debate continues. *Journal of Medical Ethics* 1996; **22**: 147-53.
2. Phillips P., Rolls B. J, Ledingham J. G. G., *et al.* Reduced thirst after water deprivation in healthy elderly men. *New England Journal of Medicine* 1984; **311:** 753-9.

3. Bevilacqua M., Norbiato G., Righini V., *et al.* Loss of osmotic thirst in multiple system atrophy: association with sinoaortic baroreceptor deafferentation. *American Journal of Physiology* 1994:**266**:1752-8.
4. Aziz L., Forsling M. L., Woolf C.. J.. The effect of intracerebroventricular injections of morphine on vasopressin release in the rat *Journal of Physiology* 1981: **311:** 401-9.
5. Craig G. M. Prostaglandins, possible mediators of the effects of oestrogen on luteinizing hormone output. *Medical Hypotheses* 1976; **2**: 116-20 (references 61-65).

DR GILLIAN CRAIG.
Northampton. 1996.

In the next chapter the focus moves from academic discussion to clinical practice. All the patients described were treated in the United Kingdom, some in hospices, others on geriatric wards, and one in a nursing home. The case reports are based on first-hand reliable information from the relatives or medical staff concerned. The scenarios described could be replicated in hospitals and hospices in other parts of the world.

Chapter 6

Some Case Studies

I'll tell you shall I, something I remember?
Something that still means a great deal to me.
It was a long time ago . . .

Eleanor Farjeon [1]

Introduction

This chapter brings to life the human tragedies behind the ethical debate. Decisions to withdraw or withhold artificial hydration and nutrition from the dying, and those who are terminally ill, have profound implications, not only for the patients, but also for their family and friends. Yet in our computer dominated society, as John Habgood has observed, personal feelings and attempts to express personal feelings tend to be regarded "as purely individual, mere matters of private opinion, not part of the real world of shared public knowledge." This trend must be resisted, said Habgood ..."we must not extinguish the value of personal experience." [2] In response to such comments some case reports are presented in the public interest to add weight to the debate and bring it to life. Statistics, which are so much easier to handle, have been described as "people with the tears washed off." [3] Tears can be dried but the reasons for the tears should not be forgotten.

Most of the cases described came to light because of conflict between doctors and relatives on the subject of hydration. Several of the patients died after six or more days without fluids. The facts of the matter have been checked wherever possible. Many of the relatives involved were devastated by their experience and suffered long term psychological distress. No one will ever know what suffering the patients endured. The cases highlight the need for empathy, sensitivity and human understanding in the management of the terminally ill.

The chapter includes some suggestions about how communication between doctors and relatives could be improved, and an analysis of the causes of failures in communication. In some cases the long-term emotional distress experienced by relatives appeared to fit the criteria for post-traumatic stress disorder.

A. Illustrative case reports

Case 1 Terminal delirium.
Case 2 Devastating stroke
Case 3 Severe pain
Case 4 Starvation in a hospital
Case 5 A life prolonged by hydration.
Case 6 An elderly patient who survived

Case 1 Terminal delirium

Terminal delirium is a situation in which parenteral sedation (that is sedation given by injection or infusion) may be required. Good management is well described in an article by Macleod, who notes that delirium is often misdiagnosed. There are many underlying causes in patients with advanced malignancy, and in 50% of cases the precise cause may not be known. Macleod observes that the presence of a near relative is important in management, adding "the family deserve and benefit from explanation, support and guidance regarding the relative's mental state." [4] Sadly such support is not always given as the following case history demonstrates.

A middle-aged man with terminal cancer and a history of mental illness was cared for in a hospice for the last few months of his life. He was not an easy man to cope with, but the hospice staff gained his trust and treated him very kindly. He could not walk in the final months and was wheel chair bound, but this did not prevent him from living life to the full, within the limitations of his physical state. His pain was controlled with morphine and his psychosis was controlled by standard anti-psychotic medication given through a syringe driver. He remained calm and brave for several months while awaiting death, but found it "a kind of torture" to be surrounded by so many dying patients. He coped largely by denial and hoped for a cure, but with the passage of time death became rather too insistent and could no longer be ignored.

Towards the end of his life his anti-psychotic medication was changed to oral chlorpromazine as the syringe driver needle was causing wheals. Thereafter, his mental state deteriorated and he became quietly psychotic. One evening a close relative visited and warned the resident doctor that all was not well, so the dose of chlorpromazine was increased. The following day there was a mental crisis. The hospice doctors telephoned the psychiatric department for advice and controlled the situation with heavy sedation that sent the patient into a deep stuporous sleep. Later that night a nurse phoned a relative who was out of town to say that the patient had "had difficulty sleeping, but now we have got him really, really comfortable, and he is not going to wake up." In response to this disturbing message the relative drove through the night to the bedside, arriving tired and worried. After talking quietly to the night nurse she went home to rest, leaving another member of the family to talk to the medical team. A few days later the first relative asked that sedation be reduced. A secret case conference was arranged, after which the junior doctor returned to the bedside and whispered that the doctors advised against reducing the main sedation, but agreed to reduce extra valium on a trial basis.

Following the reduction in valium the patient woke from his stupor and became aware of his surroundings and his visitors. He was calm again, and the delusions had gone, but he was still too sleepy or weak to drink. Over the course of the next few days, the relatives became increasingly concerned about thirst and dehydration. His life could have been prolonged with a drip, but when the need for a drip was raised the doctor in charge adamantly refused to use one. The futile telephone conversation ended with the comment "If you don't like our management take him elsewhere!" The dissenting relative had already considered this possibility and ruled it out as impracticable. There was no one local to turn to for a second opinion and no ethics committee to discuss the issues. The family had liased with professionals to good effect in the past, but on this occasion there was an impasse. To be powerless to help him at the end of life was devastating. Realising that there was nothing more they could do, they lit a candle and filled the side ward with the scent of lavender, creating a peaceful sanctuary for the patient. His last words were "Help me!" - but the family could only comfort him with their presence and love. He died peacefully, but severely dehydrated, after at least seven days of sedation without hydration.[5]

The diagnosis of a terminal delirium in this case was probably incorrect, since the patient became calm and rational on sedation. His delusions were explicable on the basis of fear and his pre-existing psychiatric illness, coupled with a change in medication to a regime that proved ineffective. Once the psychiatric crisis was controlled the question of hydration should have been addressed. The only mitigating medical factor in favour of non-intervention was an element of doubt as to whether the patient would have accepted a drip. No one thought to ask him! No one really knew! Years later the dissenting relative could remember every detail of the last traumatic week with painful clarity- it was a nightmare that changed the course of her life.

Moving the patient in cases of dispute has been suggested as a last resort by the American Medical Association.[6] They should think again! Dying patients should not be shifted around from place to place. It would be far better for health professionals to follow the advice given in our own National Ethical Guidelines and strive to address the concerns of relatives.[7]

There was a formal inquiry into the management of the case, but two independent palliative care consultants were of the opinion that the patient had been treated professionally and well. The dissenting relative felt that profound ethical problems had been overlooked and took matters further. Ultimately this disagreement sparked off the hydration debate in the United Kingdom.

There was a spiritual side to this case that must not be overlooked, for the patient was a deeply religious Christian. He attended services in the hospice chapel and was sustained by the rites of the Church. During the final traumatic week the patient and his family received loving support from a lay member of the hospice chaplaincy staff. The patient knew he was dying but still longed to live. Yet while waiting for death he had once confided "If Heaven awaits me I have lived too long!" Just before he died there was a deep sense of peace in the room. The thoughts and subdued whispers of relatives at the bedside turned to Heaven and the friends who would await him there. Many years later his family found some poems that he had written and discovered that thoughts of Heaven had sustained him for the final years of his life. This knowledge was a great comfort to them in their sorrow. The patient trusted in God and viewed his life as a pilgrimage towards the "Great I AM." May he rest in peace.

(Case reported with permission of the next of kin.)

Case 2 Devastating Stroke

An elderly lady collapsed in a nursing home, with a severe stroke that rendered her unconscious. After two days without fluids the family expressed concern and asked for a drip or naso-gastric tube to be used. The General Practitioner (GP) was consulted, but was of the opinion that a drip could not be used in a nursing home. The family explained that they did not want her to go into hospital, having been told that the journey might kill her. At this stage the GP raised his voice and pushed past them to book an ambulance to arrive within an hour. The ambulance was later cancelled. On the fifth day without hydration a Consultant visited, finding the patient terminally ill and likely to die within 24 hours or so. The patient died on the sixth day.

The relatives lodged a formal complaint through the National Health Service complaints procedure. Their main concern was that the GP knowingly deprived the patient of nutrition and water, and failed to make arrangements for her to be sustained in any way. They also felt that he had not communicated adequately with the family. The family believed that the patient must have suffered during the last six days of her life, because she had no fluids at all during that time. They were of the opinion that something should have been done about it, and pointed out that her management begged the question, had she died of dehydration or her stroke?

A committee duly met to hear the complaint about management. The Consultant took the view that artificial hydration would not have influenced the outcome. The GP admitted that he had failed to deal with the family properly. The committee recorded concern about his apparent lack of communication skills, but felt he had not been in breach of his terms of service. The complaint was dismissed.

Following the complaint, the Chief Executive of the Health Authority instigated a review of local practice regarding the care of stroke patients, but saw no need to make any changes.

The relatives were left with deep unease and wrote "It is very painful to witness a member of one's own family suffer death by dehydration. We will always feel remorseful for not insisting that she was transferred to hospital and put on a drip on the day she had the stroke. We just did not know what to do . . . Our main concern was that during those six days . . . when she was left in her nursing home bed without fluids, she must have suffered extreme discomfort from an acute sense of thirst." [8]

One can only hope that steps will be taken to teach GPs and nursing home staff about the value of subcutaneous fluids in a community setting.

(Case reported with permission of next of kin.)

Case 3 Severe Pain

An elderly man with cancer developed pain in his leg. He had radiotherapy to good effect but eventually the pain recurred and he was admitted to a hospice. An epidural line was set up - that is a fine tube through which drugs can be delivered into the spinal canal to numb the nerves. Diamorphine and a local anaesthetic given by this route controlled the pain and after three weeks he was discharged home in a wheelchair.

On hearing of plans for his discharge he wrote a letter full of hope and faith in the future. He said "I am now free of pain, which in itself is marvellous, as I was berserk with pain when I came in here, but of course I will still have the epidural in my back, with the magic solution constantly being pumped through . . . I will just have to see how mobile I can be - what I can't do I will have to forget and just concentrate on doing what I can manage. It will be hard, but my wife is my inspiration and we have great faith and a lot of good living to do, so guess we will get by." [9] Sadly this was not to be, for within a day or two the pain recurred and he was admitted to the hospice for the last time. He died there five weeks later.[9]

During the final month, pain control was variable, with good days and bad days. He sought reassurance that the Consultant would be able to help him if the pain got too bad, but at one stage asked for the morphine to be reduced as he was hallucinating. Eventually the infusion pump to the epidural failed and was taken for servicing for several hours. The following day his wife arrived to find "a plunger" in her husband's chest delivering a drug that she learnt later was midazolam. "Don't worry my darling", said her husband "it is only to relax me". His wife sensed otherwise and was deeply concerned, fearing a fatal outcome. She longed to rip the contraption out. Tension had developed between her and the medical staff, and communication was poor. When she visited, doctors seemed to vanish into side rooms to avoid her. She could get no answers to her questions. Her concerns about sustenance were ignored.

Visiting became increasingly difficult and extremely stressful. Husband and wife had always trusted each other implicitly and shared difficult decisions in life - but in death this was denied them. She longed to push her husband home, bed and all, along the pavement, but realised she could not cope with his problems. Instead she had to endure the situation, suppressing her mounting frenzy and despair. Gradually, as day followed day without food or water, her husband became unable to speak. He seemed to be struggling to say something and mouthed the words "I love you", before drifting into a coma. The day before he died his wife was horrified to see his tongue curled tight at the back of his throat, like a dry walnut. He died comatose and dehydrated after seven days on midazolam without hydration. The widow expressed the view that "It was murder. No two ways about it!"

The widow lives with a sense of guilt that she was unable to save her husband from the treatment. She is still tormented and heart-broken by sad memories. Six years after the event she wrote, "It was a barbaric end to his life . . . .. It is the most cruel, cruel thing to have to live with. I have never been able to grieve. I can only despair about what happened. My life has changed completely, mentally and physically. I am haunted by the experience . . . and vulnerable to any news items relating to decisions on terminating life. I still suffer from disturbed nights . . . and periods of deep depression . . . .. I will never know what he knew, how he felt, what he wanted so badly to say." [9]

The widow struggled for six or more years to get an independent opinion on her husband's case, without involving lawyers, to no avail. The National Health Service complaints procedure failed her. She raised concerns about euthanasia, but sources close to the professional team involved thought that management had been "exemplary". Medico-legal aspects were evaded. The hydration issue was ignored. Her Member of Parliament did his best to help. She appealed to the Health Service Ombudsman, and others but drew a blank. Sadly, at that time, the Ombudsman was not empowered to investigate clinical matters and did not see fit to authorise an independent opinion. The widow spoke movingly at a meeting in London in 1997 (see page 99 of this book.). Following this experience she sought legal advice and obtained legal aid.

Eventually after almost ten years of struggle and stress the widow obtained a helpful independent expert medical opinion and her questions were answered. Through all the years of struggle the widow felt held in a stranglehold by the medical profession whose influence dominated every avenue of complaint. Unfortunately legal aid was withdrawn before the case reached court so the medico-legal questions raised remain unanswered.

(Case reported with permission of the widow.)

Case 4 Starvation in a hospital. The case of Mrs X.

An 83 year old woman, who had been living with her son, suffered a stroke and was admitted semi-conscious to hospital. Within hours a 'do not resuscitate order' was issued despite the protests of her son. She was treated with subcutaneous fluids for some days, and on the 12th day was fitted with a naso-gastric tube. She was given virtually nothing but tap water through this tube until she died, seven and a half weeks after admission.

The son was aware that his mother was in danger. He tried and failed, to get her transferred elsewhere. His repeated requests that she be given nourishment were ignored. He offered to pay for the necessary nourishment, to no avail. He spoke to the dietician who deferred to the Consultant. The son and other visitors gave her sips of cranberry juice that she seemed to swallow, but of course this did not suffice.

"No words can possibly describe how it felt- " he wrote. He lost 4 stone in weight, could not sleep, and spent hours at his mother's bedside talking to her. Occasionally she spoke a word that indicated that she had heard and understood. Of course she died, for no one can survive indefinitely without food. Death was attributed to a cerebrovascular accident and hypertension. Malnutrition was not mentioned and no post-mortem was performed.

It is acceptable to provide fluids without nutrients for a few days in stroke patients who cannot swallow, or are in stupor or coma. To continue this management for a period of weeks is unacceptable in the view of the British Association for Parenteral and Enteral Nutrition as it leads to progressive malnutrition.

(Case quoted with the son's permission.)

Case 5 A life prolonged by hydration.

A young mother aged 28, with a rare tumour of the biliary tract, was determined to live. She underwent surgery to remove the primary tumour and later, at her insistence, had surgery to remove four liver metastases. One proved technically impossible to remove as it was too close to a major artery. Surgery was followed by some radiotherapy and chemotherapy. She developed pain that was difficult to control despite a coeliac plexus nerve block. A CT scan was normal, but when repeated a month later showed a large shadow, reported to be a metastasis. Yet again the patient requested surgery. At operation the 'shadow' was found to be an abscess that was drained. After a stormy post-operative course in hospital she returned to the hospice, and eventually went home again to her husband and children.

Several weeks later the hospice Consultant returned from a short holiday to find the patient back in the hospice, very weak and deteriorating. He assumed she was dying. After five days of decline she became unconscious and all her relatives arrived.

Her brother insisted that she have intravenous fluids and antibiotics, to which the Consultant agreed for the sake of the family. To his astonishment the patient steadily recovered.

When she was fully conscious he sat down with her and she asked "Why did you not give me fluids until my brother insisted"? The Consultant replied that he had thought she was dying. She asked what would have happened if her brother had not insisted and the doctor admitted that she would have died. He told her that he had made a terrible mistake and that she had nearly died of dehydration because of his error. He then debated with her whether she felt able to trust him any more. After thinking about it carefully, she and her husband told the Consultant that they could trust him and they wanted him to continue to care for herwhich he did. The patient lived for several more months, with intermittent severe pain and emotional distress. She continued to hope for a cure until the moment she died, and always wanted everything done to prolong her life. She was given intravenous antibiotics again - at her request - as she was deteriorating, but they made no difference and were stopped. In the end she died quite suddenly.

This patient will always remain a very painful memory for the doctor concerned. His only consolation was that several hospital colleagues said they would have made the same incorrect assumption. Would that all palliative carers were as honest and sensitive as that doctor!

(Case quoted with the Consultant's permission)

Case 6 An elderly patient who survived

An elderly woman living in a local authority residential home was seen on a domiciliary visit by a Consultant Geriatrician, at the request of the patient's General Practitioner (GP). She was quite disabled by arthritis and had suffered a stroke in the past. The GP had indicated to the Consultant that she did not want the patient admitted to hospital. The problems were abdominal distension with vomiting, general lethargy, weakness and constipation. On examination the patient was slightly dehydrated and had intestinal obstruction due to severe constipation (faecal impaction). This is not unusual in old people, but the diagnosis can be overlooked. The situation was explained to relatives who agreed to admission. The patient made a dramatic recovery after a successful enema and rehydration. Had she remained untreated she would have died.

(Case quoted with the Consultant's permission)

General discussion.

Undoubtedly there are times when some sedation is needed to relieve intolerable distress, but it does not necessarily follow that the patient should be allowed to develop fatal dehydration as a consequence of sedation. Note for example, that in cases 1 and 3 sedation relieved the patient's distress and both were calm, comfortable and able to talk for a while. However, as dehydration took its toll, their condition deteriorated and they died. It is questionable whether the doctrine of double effect is valid under such circumstances.

Many of the cases described in this chapter are worrying, yet relatives who complained through formal channels were given a rough ride, for it was always possible to find a senior doctor who approved of the care given. However strongly one may feel about management in an individual case, others may feel equally strongly that the patient's best interests were served. Some might think it acceptable to shorten life by withholding artificial hydration in order to prevent the possibility of future suffering, but others would disagree. There are no easy answers in medical ethics! Exceptionally difficult problems, that stretch medical skill and patience to the uttermost, do sometimes arise in palliative care.

In two of the cases reported above, severe mental distress and intolerable pain were controlled in a hospice, but at a price using sedation without hydration. Sedation *with* hydration to prevent terminal dehydration would have improved the patient's comfort and reduced the relative's distress. However taxing the clinical situation, inconsiderate behaviour towards relatives cannot be condoned. It is now acknowledged by the General Medical Council that patients and their families and others close to them should be treated with understanding and compassion.

B. Post-traumatic stress disorder

Seriously distressing life events can give rise to a syndrome known as Post-traumatic Stress Disorder (PTSD). Certain criteria have to be fulfilled before a diagnosis of PTSD can be accepted. The American Psychiatric Association Diagnostic and Statistical Manual (DSM-IV), as quoted by Dr Turner [10] requires the following objective and subjective criteria:-

i) *The person experienced, witnessed or was confronted with an event or events that involved actual or threatened death or serious injury, or a threat to the physical integrity of self or others.*
ii) *The person's response involved intense fear, helplessness or horror.*
(Note: in children this may be expressed instead by disorganised or agitated behaviour.)

The magnitude of the stress is important, as is the subjective perception of the trauma.[10] Disasters such as the fire at King's Cross Underground Station in London caused PTSD in survivors. However, policemen involved in the Hillsborough football stadium disaster, when many spectators were crushed to death, were not allowed to claim for damages for PTSD, as the stress was encountered in the course of their normal occupation.

The adverse psychological reactions reported by some relatives in cases 1 - 4 of the preceding section are summarised in Table 1. With the exception of guilt, they tally with the symptoms of PTSD as described by Turner.[10] The relatives were witness to a traumatic event as defined in DSM-IV. They experienced anguish and were helpless to intervene in the face of a threat to the physical integrity of their loved ones. They were adversely affected by their experience and suffered long term psychological symptoms. All relatives were intensely aware that hydration and/or nutritional needs were not being met.

Table 1 Symptoms experienced by relatives

- Guilt and remorse
- Depression
- Hyperarousal and anxiety
- Persisting psychological difficulties
- Avoidance behaviour
- Pressure on relationships
- Intrusive thoughts and flashbacks
- Long term anger and struggle

A sense of guilt was expressed by all the relatives. Most felt guilty for not being more forceful in their efforts to persuade doctors to use artificial hydration. It is fair to say however, that no amount of persuasion is likely to influence a doctor whose mind is set on non-intervention. Even medically qualified relatives are in a weak negotiating position when not professionally involved in patient care. Relatives have no standing in law at present in England and Wales. However in countries where relatives or friends can be lawfully appointed as proxy health care decision-makers (for example, Scotland and the USA), their views have to be heeded by doctors.

Anguish of responsibility. Some relatives felt that they had betrayed their loved ones by putting them in a position where they could die of dehydration. In cases 1 and 3 the relatives considered moving the patient from the hospice but realised this was futile. "He trusted me" said one "and look what happened!" They were shocked by their experience. The distress experienced by those who care for the dying has been described as an anguish of responsibility, or a torment of responsibility rather than guilt, when experienced by professional carers, i.e. doctors or nurses. "The torment of responsibility develops into a deeper existential anguish, thus linking up with the patient's moral or spiritual suffering" writes Dr Marie Frings.[11] This anguish or guilt, call it what you will, can undoubtedly affect close relatives too.

Depression was common and some people felt suicidal at times. Intense distrust of the medical profession made it difficult for one woman to accept help.

Hyperarousal and intense anxiety caused sleep disturbance, anger, or an intense reaction to news items as described by the relative in case 3. Some people affected by PTSD resort to self-medication with alcohol to reduce anxiety. One woman needed beta blockers for tachycardia during the final days with her dying relative; another fortified herself with brandy.

Persisting psychological difficulties. The longterm adverse effects of PTSD can last for many years. There is evidence that noradrenaline, a neurotransmitter released from sympathetic nerve endings during stress, can etch memories into the brain, and cause retention of distressing and highly arousing memories through an effect on the amygdala. This was reported by Dr Ronan O'Carroll at the British Psychological Society in 1998.[12]

Avoidance behaviour. Affected relatives tend to avoid people and places that remind them of the traumatic incident. Where the relative is a doctor or nurse, post-traumatic stress provoked by experiences such as those described can make it difficult to continue to work. This is yet another reason for treating such relatives with great sensitivity. Sadly the art of involving knowledgeable relatives in end-of-life decisions has yet to be learnt by the majority of doctors.

Pressure on relationships. Sometimes different members of a family have different views on medical ethics. Those who feel strongly about the need for hydration may not be supported in their views by the others, and vice versa. This can cause problems within families.

Intrusive thoughts and flashbacks. People affected by PTSD may relive the traumatic experience unexpectedly, sometimes in the early hours of the morning, or when low spirited in the day. Flashbacks can be caused by news, chance remarks, or anything that reminds the person of the event.

Long term anger and struggle. Anger or a sense of injustice may motivate relatives who resolve to improve the situation. Constructive anger helps individuals to cope, and changes situations for the better. Slowly but surely with courage and determination, relatives all over the country are making their voices heard in the corridors of power.

In conclusion.

My opinion that the symptoms experienced by some relatives amounted to PTSD is based on personal insight, empathy, conversations and correspondence with the people concerned. Psychologists might entertain alternative diagnoses, such as bereavement reaction for example. Some comments made by John Habgood are relevant. He said "to understand another person's actions or feelings by empathy with them, is to have a different kind of knowledge from that of the psychologist or sociologist . . . The different levels of understanding can reinforce one another . . . Which most entitles us to say that we 'know' that other person however, psychological categorisation or personal insight?" [13]

The psychological label has therapeutic and medico-legal significance. However, setting formal categorisation aside, the important point for people to grasp is that the experience of seeing a loved one die of dehydration or starvation before your eyes, when medical staff refuse to intervene is absolutely devastating. It can destroy lives by causing long term psychological damage and distress. It is totally unacceptable that relatives should suffer in this way at the hands of the medical profession.

While writing this chapter, I was struck by a sentence in a book review in The Times. The book, about the First World War, was '1915: The Death of Innocence' by Lyn Macdonald. The reviewer wrote 'Macdonald has, without sentimentality or anger, allowed those of us who were there to remind those of us who were not, that we should see it through their eyes or forever misunderstand' [14]. *This* chapter, indeed *this book* 'No Water: No Life', is about the death of innocence too – the death of innocent patients, the death of trust in the medical profession. We must see this through the eyes of the relatives who were there or forever misunderstand. Some will carry their dismay and grief to the grave. For them the long and dusty road of painful memories seems to have no end.

> "I dragged on the dusty road, and I remember
> How the old woman looked over the fence at me
> and seemed to know how it felt . . .
> . . . the long dusty road seemed to have for me
> No end, you know."
>
> *Eleanor Farjeon* [1]

C. Addressing the anxieties of relatives

In the course of the debate in the Journal of Medical Ethics, Dunlop et al agreed that there are times when it is justifiable to give subcutaneous fluids for the sake of the family.[15] Dunphy et al went further and stressed the need "above all to be responsive to the wishes of the family." [16] Current professional guidelines for palliative carers states- "Relatives at the bedside of dying patients frequently express concern about lack of fluid or nutrition intake. Health care professionals may not subordinate the interests of patients to the anxieties of relatives, but should nevertheless strive to address those anxieties." [7]

Advice on addressing the anxieties of relatives.

C1. *Listen carefully* and do not dismiss the views given; everyone with genuine concerns deserves to be heard. Relatives may have valid and important observations to make. They will have known the patient for much longer than the health care professionals involved.

C2. *Give relatives time*: choose the right moment to approach them. Do not expect them to talk when tired and distressed and then label them 'difficult to access', if they decline. If they approach you, try to set aside a mutually convenient time and place to talk. Don't forget that most relatives who work have to visit in the evening or at the weekend. Someone other than the most junior member of staff should be available to talk to them.

C3. *Acknowledge professional expertise* when it is present, even if the views expressed do not tally with your own. There are two sides to every story. It may be particularly important to discuss issues with medically qualified relatives who understand better than most what is going on. Trained observers in the role of relatives cannot switch off professionally and become all accepting, submissive, uninformed members of the public, to order. It simply cannot be done - nor should it be expected when serious ethical issues are at stake.

C4. *Include concerned relatives in discussions*- unless they do not want to be involved.
- There must be a suitable forum for debate. Secret case conferences behind closed doors are simply not acceptable.
- Transfer of the patient to a hospice or hospital will not eliminate the relatives' need to be involved in many cases, although some will be only too thankful to hand over completely to the professionals.

C5. *Always be courteous.* Do not swear or thump the table! Do not be hostile to those who disagree with you.

C6. *Do not take confidentiality to extremes* as this can have adverse consequences. Although relatives have no standing in law in medical decisions in the UK at present, there are times when they should be involved. They may be the main carer of frail and vulnerable people, entrusted with medication and other personal matters.

C7. *The child/parent roles* are sometimes reversed at the end of life and this should be recognised by health care professionals. Dr John Wyatt, a paediatrician, considers that providing terminal care for a severely handicapped infant is "not different in kind from providing terminal care to a dying elderly patient".[17] He treats the parents with great sensitivity and includes them in full and adequate discussion about medical recommendations to withdraw care. I believe that the relatives of dying adult patients should be treated with equal sensitivity and respect.

C8. *Recognise the skills of relatives* I once observed a man visiting his wife in hospital. She was on chronic peritoneal dialysis and had been admitted to hospital for assessment. He normally coped with her dialysis at home - but now felt that his role had been usurped by the doctors. He was hurt, angry, unhappy, even a little jealous, and definitely ill at ease with the way things were being done. The doctors concerned were unaware of this and carried on regardless, while marital harmony deteriorated.

C9. *Be sensitive to couples.* Crucial decisions regarding a spouse or partner should be taken jointly if possible. There may however, be times when one partner may try to protect the other from painful reality. This is well recognised when it comes to sharing knowledge of a fatal diagnosis, and most people feel that an open attitude is best. It is possible to envisage a similar situation arising at the end of life. The struggle to endure pain or distress may be too great, and the need to give up too painful to mention to a loved one. Such situations, if recognised, should be approached with great gentleness and sensitivity.

C10. *When serious distress arises*, the medical profession should act to limit the psychological damage to relatives. It is not sufficient to wave them goodbye and leave them to sink or swim alone.

A three-point approach is recommended by Dr Stuart Turner, an expert on Post-traumatic Stress Disorder (PTSD).[10]

- *Firstly* Apologise and explain the situation honestly.
- *Secondly* Arrange skilled psychological debriefing within a few days of the event, by professionally trained and experienced people. This may help to reduce distress, improve the ability to copy, and may even prevent PTSD.
- *Thirdly* For those who develop longer-term reactions, there are now effective interventions, and early referral for specialist treatment may be appropriate.[10]

I would add a reminder that in a hospice or hospital setting many relatives will have travelled from a distance. If they are distressed it would be advisable to suggest that they contact their own doctor. Offer to write a letter to the doctor if need be.

C11. *A duty to care is a duty to listen.* Professor Ilora Finlay, speaking at a conference at the Royal College of Physicians in March 1999 stressed the need for sincere human empathy when talking to relatives. She observed that the range of families encountered is wide. Some are loving, some give mixed messages, others could be described as families from hell. Some individuals who appear uninvolved, with an air of quiet efficiency, may be difficult to communicate with, according to Professor Finlay. She quoted published evidence that 23% of bereaved relatives had no discussion, and 44% wanted better communication in a hospice setting. There may also be unsatisfactory communication between couples, or within families, as people try to protect each other from painful reality.[18]

"The duty to care is a duty to listen," said Professor Finlay - adding "but listen to whom? The patient, next of kin, children, other professionals, or friends?" The relative can be regarded as a secondary patient, and suffering psychological trauma - indeed, the whole family is the patient, in the view of Professor Finlay. There may be inherent tension between the needs of the patient and the needs of the family.[18] In the course of discussion, Professor Finlay stressed that doctors must engage relatives in care in a positive way and be more honest. We must also bear in mind that discussion, of risks and benefits for example, may be a great burden to relatives.[18]

This sensitive approach to relatives was not shared by a doctor who told conference delegates how she had responded to a relative who disagreed with her management. "Would your attitude change if I returned with my lawyer?" the relative asked - to which the doctor replied "No!". This response is in keeping with the view that "It is no more defensible to provide or omit a drip purely on the basis of the wishes of the relative, than it is on the basis of the culture of the admitting unit, or on the contents of its written philosophy." [19] Yet in their book on Palliative Care Ethics, Randall and Downie talk about the common humanity of doctor and patient.[20] Perhaps some doctors have yet to learn that relatives are human too!

In summary Key relatives need to be involved, honestly, openly and with compassion. If they are badly treated by the medical profession they may become patients too, and suffer long-term psychological distress.

D. When communication fails

I would now like to consider some of the causes of communication failure between doctors and relatives, in the hope of shedding light on the situation.

D1. Some doctors seem reluctant to engage in serious discussion with relatives. They appear to avoid them and leave it to others to pass on important decisions. Others meet hurriedly and depart speedily, leaving distrust in their wake. After one unsatisfactory encounter relatives may avoid the doctor concerned, finding further discussion futile. The BMA advise that relatives should be involved in discussions and decisions about withholding life-prolonging treatment, yet discussion may be rendered futile by the entrenched views of the health care team, or relatives. Either way there may be an impasse.

D2. Some health care staff try to protect relatives from painful reality. This approach is perfectly valid but should not be taken to extremes. It should be possible to convey the truth with gentleness and honesty. There is an art in communicating bad news.

D3. Corner and Dunlop writing in 'New Themes in Palliative Care', mentioned the work of McNamara.[21] He found that a 'good death' can be 'required' by hospice staff. Patients 'who did not conform to this ideal . . . by hanging on to life, were felt to have 'problems'.[22] Presumably dissenting relatives who request life-prolonging treatment for their loved ones may also be perceived to have problems, or to be a problem to the staff. On occasions, staff will employ subterfuge and deceit to achieve their ends. The death-orientated approach has to prevail in such institutions. Thus relatives who ask for a drip to be used may be seen as a major threat by hospice staff. Such relatives have to overcome the prejudice of a whole institutionalised system. That is a lot to ask of an emotionally drained, grieving individual. Those who fail should certainly not blame themselves.

D4. Health care professionals may reach the end of their emotional and professional resources when caring for distressing cases. There is then a risk that patients may be sedated inappropriately, as Main observed years ago.[23] Doctors may find themselves under pressure from nursing staff to "do something" to end the situation. If this happens a wise doctor will seek a second opinion, but medical pride and the autonomy of the institution can sometimes stand in the way of wisdom.

The British Medical Association now recommend additional safeguards and a second opinion, before artificial hydration or nutrition is withdrawn from patients who are not terminally ill.[24] Unfortunately neither the BMA nor General Medical Council [25] insist that this safeguard be extended to patients who are dying.

D5. Main, who drew attention to the problem of inappropriate sedation, also reported that certain patients have a strange influence on carers [23] with the result that some carers feel they are the only people who understand the patient. Staff with this view could come into conflict with relatives who also hold this view, but whose opinions about appropriate action differ. Thus there may be opposing views about the patient's "best interest".

D6. Health care professionals must be careful not to substitute their own interests for those of the patient. Thus concerns about pressure on beds, or resentment about caring for elderly 'bed blockers' must not be allowed to influence clinical judgement.

D7. Abrupt behaviour is sometimes an expression of strong emotions. If your professional view as to what is right and proper is questioned, it may be difficult to cope with the situation. Some people pull rank, others adopt a 'take it or leave it' stance - yet others rush out of the room, or show people the door. It would be preferable to sit down quietly and discuss the situation.

D8. The setting in which a patient is cared for, and the skills and attitudes of the carers, can dictate the level of care as Dunphy and colleagues observed.[16] This is extremely important to recognise especially in the care of the dying. It is now recognised in national guidelines that "the practicalities of appropriate provision will vary according to the setting, but good practice will require that patients needing artificial hydration are transferred to a unit equipped to provide such care".[7] An evaluation of the burdens and benefits of intervention should include an assessment of whether the patient would wish to be moved, or should be moved to a setting that can provide a higher level of care. Decisions should be made by gentle discussion with those concerned. Wider provision of subcutaneous hydration in community settings would spare many patients a last minute, undignified and disturbing move to hospital.

D9. In tight-knit units, staff may be reluctant to hand the patient over to another team. There is an emotional investment in providing care and a natural wish to see the patient through to the end. Moves can be disruptive. So undue pressure one way or another can lead to conflict. Decisions must be made with the patient's best interest at heart, not for the emotional satisfaction of the staff. Yet one should consider the staff and try to avoid severing caring bonds unnecessarily. All these factors have to be considered when weighing up the pros and cons of transferring the patient elsewhere. It is sad for all concerned when relations between staff and relatives break down, for at base, all have - or should have - the patient's best interest at heart.

D10. Relatives who meet a Consultant who is sympathetic and willing to listen are fortunate. They may be spared the agony that others experience. In our overstretched health service, it is often difficult for doctors to spend adequate time with their patients, let alone with relatives. Therefore discussion if it occurs at all, is likely to be hurried. There should be designated staff whose role is to ease situations of conflict. A few medical ethicists are now in post in the UK, and in the USA consultation-liaison psychiatrists are proving helpful in medical futility situations.[26]

D11. Health care professionals as relatives may be in a particularly difficult situation. Their professional expertise should be recognised. This is not the same as asking, or expecting them to be clinically involved, but it does mean that there should be an appropriate level of discussion of clinical matters when necessary. Professional relatives will inevitably take an interest in clinical matters, and may find the enforced change of role to that of a relative difficult.

Most doctors are very conscious of the need not to intrude with their own views unless this seems essential. Sometimes it is essential. It may be that they have made an observation that needs to be passed on. Maybe they disagree with the diagnosis, maybe they would approach the problem in an entirely different way. If so, they should make their views known quietly. Suggestions made quietly by a colleague should be taken seriously. We don't all jump up and down or shout! There is an art in coping with medical relatives. A little bit of professional courtesy goes a long way and will ease the most difficult situations.

An excellent example of how matters should be handled was shown in a BBC television drama series about medical ethics. The series, called 'Life Support' was broadcast in the summer of 1999.[27] In the final episode, the medical ethicist was asked to make the most difficult decision of her life. She found herself in the role of a relative, as her father lay dying in the Coronary Care Unit after a massive heart attack. There was nothing more that could be done and the time had come to wean him off cardiac stimulants and oxygen. The consultant in charge sought her out, spoke to her gently, reminded her that she was not there as a doctor and that it was time to let the dying man go. He then explained what the approach would be. Colleagues supported her and recognised her emotional needs. That is how it should be done!

D12. Relatives can be unreasonable. Their views may be inappropriate, dangerous, or not in the patient's best interest. Sometimes a doctor cannot accede to them and maintain professional integrity. Relatives are not always well disposed towards the patient, nor are they necessarily good advocates. Some may have reason to wish the patient dead- they may want to take over their house, inherit their money or marry their spouse! Many hidden agendas influence decision- making. Health care professionals and others need to be aware of these dangers.

Consider the folllowing scenaria. An elderly lady was persuaded by her daughter to go home, rather than into a nursing home, even though she was not capable of looking after herself. The patient was considered to be *compos mentis*. The health care team seemed to be unaware that finance was available to fund nursing care. The patient was discharged home with inadequate support, fell over within a week, was readmitted to hospital and died. The daughter gained her inheritance. The doctors learnt a hard lesson about human nature.

Occasionally relatives will go so far as to threaten a doctor with physical harm if treatment is withdrawn. A case of such blackmail was reported recently.[28] Sometimes a group of relatives and neighbours confront doctors with their views as to what should be done. Sometimes their views are heeded to good effect, sometimes their views are not welcome, and it has been known for a fracas to develop as happened in the case of David Glass.[29] Such events are fortunately rare, and should be avoidable if doctors act with sensitivity.

Some relatives find the thought of artificial hydration and nutrition abhorrent, or frightening. "All those tubes - are they really necessary? Wouldn't it be kinder to let her go?" They may not understand that the medical situation could improve. Patients must not be abandoned to their fate, if recovery is possible, simply because relatives find it painful to look at a drip or feeding tube. It may be distressing to see a loved one dependent on technology, but it is worth enduring such distress for the sake of the patient. An irrational, Luddite opposition to technology is not helpful in medicine. The art is to know how to employ technology at the optimal level, using the simplest method that will achieve the benefit sought. Careful analysis of the risks and benefits by qualified medical staff, with relatives if appropriate, is essential.

Summary

Many difficulties in communication in medical practice arise from a lack of compassion. Intellectual analysis of clinical problems, though essential, can get in the way of empathy. There may be a determination on the part of doctors to do things their way, a failure to be sensitive to the needs of others who see things rather differently. Doctors and nurses may fail to hear a cry for help casually expressed, may fail to consider the wishes of the patient or their family. Good communication with relatives is vital under all circumstances.

Causes of communication break down
- Poor communication skills
- Lack of empathy
- Lack of compassion
- Lack of time
- Relatives seen as a threat
- Death 'required' of patient
- Patient characteristics [23]
- Lack of knowledge or experience
- Over emphasis on confidentiality
- Negligence
- Autonomy of health care team.
- Rivalry and wish to dominate
- Rudeness, anger or arrogance
- Tiredness and stress
- Unreasonable demands from relatives

Jean Vanier, a French philosopher, has written about the need to rediscover a common humanity in our dealings with other people. It is too easy to hide behind walls of poor communication. "Real communication is difficult" wrote Vanier – "It implies a choice, commitment, gentleness, trust and respect for the other...."[30] Clearly a doctor's main responsibility is to the patient, but wise doctors now recognise that they also have a responsibility to the patient's family.

Sheppard and Warlock, senior clergy working in Liverpool in the 1980s, noted that a strong sense of identity between groups of people can lead to a kind of tribalism, 'a retreat into a fortress mentality that is closed to any argument or explanation if it seems to threaten tribal customs. Then the quick wit ceases to be good-humoured and develops an aggressive defensive tone, keeping strangers at arm's length'.[31] Within the Health Service, this can affect doctor/patient relationships, and communication between health care staff and relatives. A fortress mentality can also impede communication between doctors working in different specialties such as palliative care and geriatric medicine. We must all strive to find our common humanity, pocket our pride, and put the interests of our patients first.

References

1. Farjeon E H. It was a long time ago. Page 83 in Tapestry, an anthology. (c)Eric Williams. *Arnold* 1974.
2. Habgood J. Being a person. Ch. 8, Words and thoughts. p.167. *Hodder & Stoughton,* 1998.
3. Sidel V W. A quote from *The Lancet.* 1985; 7th Dec. p.1287-1289.
4. Macleod A D. The clinical management of delirium in hospice practice. *European Journal of Palliative Care.* 1997; **4**: 116-120.
5. Case quoted with permission of next-of-kin.
6. Charaton F. AMA issues guidelines on end of life care. *British Medical Journal.* 1999; **318**: 690.
7. Artificial hydration (AH) for people who are terminally ill. *National Council for Hospice and Specialist Palliative Care Services* 1997.
8. Wise P. Personal communication, quoted with permission.
9. Quoted with the permission of the widow.
10. Turner S. Post-Traumatic Stress Disorder. *Journal of the Medical and Dental Defence Unions.* 1995;11: 32-33. (c) MDU, 1995. All rights reserved.
11. Frings M. Palliative care and the need for a metaphysical approach. European Journal of Palliative Care. 1997; 4(4): 129-132.
12. O'Carroll R. E, Drysdale E, Cahill L, Shajahan P, Ebmeier K P. Stimulation of the noradrenergic system enhances, and blockade reduces memory for emotional material in man. *Psychological Medicine.* 1999; **29**: part 1, p105-112.
13. Habgood J. In God's image. Chapter 10. p.216-7 in "Being a person". *Hodder & Stoughton.* 1998.
14. Macdonald Lyn. "1915: the Death of Innocence." *Headline.* 1997.
15. Dunlop RJ, Ellershaw JE, Baines HJ, Sykes N, Saunders M. Journal of Medical Ethics. 1995; **21**: 141-143.
16. Dunphy K, Finlay I, Rathbone G, Gilbert J, Hicks F. Rehydration in palliative and terminal care: if not-why not? *Palliative Medicine* 1995; **9**: 221-228.
17. Wyatt J. Treatment decisions regarding the severely handicapped newborn. In 'A Time to Die'. *CBPP.* London, 1997.

18. Finlay I. Talking to relatives. Paper given at Royal College of Physicians of London. March 24th 1999.

19. Dunphy K and Randall F. Ethical decision making in palliative care. *European Journal of Palliative Care*. 1997; **4**: 126-128

20. Randall F and Downie R. Palliative Care Ethics. *Oxford University Press*. 1996; p.152

21. Corner J, Dunlop R. New approaches to care. Ch. 18, p.289 in New Themes in Palliative Care. Ed. Clark D, Hockley J, Ahmedzai S. *Open University Press*. 1997.

22. McNamara B, Waddell C and Colvin M. The institutionalisation of the good death. *Social Science and Medicine*. 1994; **39**: (11): 1501-8. Quoted by Corner & Dunlop.

23. Main T F. The ailment. *British Journal of Medical Psychology*. 1957; **30**: 129-145.

24. Withholding and withdrawing Life-Prolonging Medical Treatment, Guidance for decision making. British Medical Association, June 1999.

25. Withholding and Withdrawing Life-prolonging Treatments: Good Practice in Decision-making. General Medical Council, London, August 2002.

26. Strain J, Snyder S, Drooker M. Conflict resolution: experience of consultation-liaison psychiatrists. Chapter 10. p.98-109 in Medical Futility. *Cambridge University Press*. 1997.

27. 'Life support' BBC Television 1999. Written by Ashley Pharoah; Director, Morag Fullarton; Professional Adviser, Dr. David Cook.

28. Knetch J (a pseudonym). At the coalface: medical ethics in practice: "He is too young to die . . . and you too, doctor". *Journal of Medical Ethics*. 1999; **25**: 418.

29. Badly treated. Leading article (anon). The Daily Telegraph. July 17th 2000, p.21.

30. Vanier J. The thirst for communion. p.50 in "Our Journey Home." *Hodder & Stoughton* 1997.

31. Sheppard D and Warlock D. p.42 in "Better Together". *Hodder & Stoughton* 1988.

(Note: A shorter version of this chapter was first submitted for publication in 1999.)
© Craig 1999

Chapter 7

A Geriatrician's Perspective

Palliative care from the perspective of a Consultant Geriatrician: the dangers of withholding hydration

Gillian Craig, MD, FRCP

Reprinted from Ethics & Medicine (1999) 15:1,15—19

Abstract

Dr Craig reviews arguments she put forward in a paper in the Journal of Medical Ethics in 1994.[1] This became the focus for wide debate of the ethical and legal dilemmas that arise when hydration is withheld in terminally ill patients. As a result national guidelines on the ethical use of artificial hydration were developed.[2]

Sedation without hydration is dangerous on medical, physiological, ethical and legal grounds, and can be disturbing for relatives. Doctors are fallible, and diagnostic errors not uncommon. Doctors are legally responsible for their acts and their omissions and must not abuse their power. Attention to hydration is not merely optional, it should be a basic part of good medicine and good palliative care.

Recommendations made by Dr. Craig in 1997.
There should be:
- An obligatory second Consultant opinion when sedation without hydration is considered.
- A confidential enquiry into the use of parenteral sedation in palliative care, and some effective monitoring system.
- A forum for resolving clinical ethical disputes during life.
- Research into thirst perception in the dying.
- A life-orientated approach to palliative care, in keeping with the best traditions of the hospice movement.

The dangers of withholding hydration

As a geriatrician I cared for many dying patients on my wards, but geriatrics is not primarily about death and dying. It is about supporting frail people in the last years of life. A holistic approach is essential, therapeutic nihilism is not. 'Our task'—to quote Professor Millard—'is not to accelerate death, but to care.' Another geriatrician Professor Sir John Grimley Evans, has spoken of the need for correct compassion.

Attention to hydration was routine on my wards, and drips were used when necessary. It would have been inconceivable for my team to have deliberately allowed a patient to die of dehydration. I was therefore shocked to discover the intensity of opposition to drips in the hospice movement a few years ago, when it was as futile to ask for a drip as to ask the incoming tide to turn. I criticised this attitude in a paper in the journal of Medical Ethics that became a focus for debate, leading to the publication of national ethical guidelines on the use of artificial hydration in terminally ill patients [2] It is now acknowledged that a rigid policy for or against artificial hydration in terminal care is ethically indefensible. The aim now is to encourage palliative carers to make patient-centred decisions, weighing up the potential benefits and burdens of intervention. So at last the tide is turning. Much progress has been made, for which I thank all concerned.

There are times in palliative care when a drip is not necessary, even when a patient cannot drink, for example if the patient is overhydrated or in heart failure. Some patients die suddenly without becoming dehydrated, so the problem of maintaining hydration does not arise. However, a rigid antagonism to artificial hydration under all circumstances in the dying is dangerous. I know of cancer patients who have been sedated and left without fluids or nourishment for over a week until they died, grossly dehydrated, despite the protests of their relatives. To watch a loved one die in this way is profoundly disturbing and can cause post traumatic stress. Yet I realise that some people who specialise in palliative medicine see prolongation of life as undesirable, even meddlesome, a mere prolongation of the dying process. This may explain much of the reluctance to use drips. If death is seen as a welcome relief, it is convenient to regard hydration as optional, rather than obligatory. Convenient, but morally debatable. There is a view that is shared by many thoughtful people, that hydration and nutrition are basic human needs, and should not be regarded as treatment that a doctor may give or withhold. In my opinion attention to hydration is not merely optional, it should be a basic part of good medicine and good palliative care.

Withholding hydration is dangerous on medical, ethical and legal grounds. It may shorten the life of patients, add to their distress, and cause their relatives anguish.

First the medical dangers

Doctors are fallible. Patients referred for terminal care may not be terminally ill. They may have been misdiagnosed. They may have a treatable complication such as sepsis after surgery for cancer, or diabetes associated with cancer of the pancreas. Small liver lesions can be mistaken for cancer deposits on ultrasounds or scans, and so on. Accurate histological diagnosis is also essential. One doctor reported a patient who is alive and well seven years after being written off with extensive malignant disease. A last ditch biopsy showed a type of tumour that responded to chemotherapy.[3] As Dr Caplan of the Hastings Centre once put it – "The new era of diagnostic paraphernalia has brought about a shift, not in the overall rate of diagnostic error, but in the type of error that is made."

A rigorous post-mortem study published in the Journal of Pathology in 1981 showed that in 39% of over 1000 hospital autopsies, the main clinical diagnosis was not confirmed, or was only a subsidiary cause of death.[4] In half of these cases a different treatment would have been given had the correct diagnosis been known. Diagnostic errors rose from 22% in the under 45s, to 53% in the over 75s. In 1981 16% of patients who were thought to have died of malignancy had died of something else, such as infections or clots in the lungs. The Royal Colleges Working Party Report of 1991 quotes a figure of 25%,[50] so there is cause for concern and humility. Doctors must be absolutely sure of the diagnosis before making irreversible treatment limiting decisions. Many people could die for want of a drip.

A closer look at patients dying of a terminal confusional state might uncover a plethora of treatable conditions, yet treatment by sedation without hydration is thought to be acceptable. Any confusional state treated in this way will prove terminal. And what about the problem of intractable pain? Is infusion of midazolam and morphine without hydration for days on end until death occurs, really an acceptable solution? Is it really acceptable that such treatment can be given on the word of one doctor or a hospice team, without the patient's truly informed consent, and without prior discussion with the next of kin? How would you feel if it was your husband, or your wife lying there, unable to speak, the last goodbyes unsaid? I think you would feel shocked and betrayed. It would be like a nightmare.[6]

Society has spent much time considering the ethics of withdrawing hydration and nourishment from patients in a permanent vegetative state. Surely equally careful attention should be given to hydration in the dying. When sedation without hydration is considered for any reason a second Consultant opinion should be obligatory, for 'Consultants are as likely as anyone else to make mistakes or err in judgement'.[7] I would like to see a confidential enquiry into the use of parenteral sedation in palliative care, and some effective monitoring system.

Sometimes fluids are withheld by doctors who genuinely feel that treatment is futile or the quality of life too poor, or even that the burden on relatives is too great. This is a danger area, not only for cancer patients, but also for elderly stroke patients, who are sometimes left to die untreated, and incompletely diagnosed, although conscious and aware. Yet they, like many hospice patients, may find life worthwhile and precious despite their frailty. It is unethical to deny such people life by withholding hydration.

If a patient cannot speak for himself, it is good practice to ask the relatives what the patient's views about treatment might be, but relatives have no standing in law in such matters in the UK. Also the well being of the patient must not be compromised for the sake of relatives—or indeed health care staff, whose response to a difficult situation may be to wish the patient dead and out of misery.

No one should be forced to watch a loved one die while doctors refuse to give fluids, but sadly such cases still arise. It is not widely known that subcutaneous fluids can be given in a community setting. Not so long ago a woman watched her sister die in a nursing home after a severe brain stem stroke. She lay for six days without fluids, although the sister asked for a drip and agonised about thirst. A drip would probably not have altered the fatal outcome for the patient, but it would have spared the relative intense distress. Never underestimate the pain that such relatives suffer. Do not ignore their views or exclude them from discussions. If you do they may never recover from the experience. It is our job as doctors to ensure that the family can go on living, without being haunted by the manner of their loved one's death.

Society must address the issue of how best to resolve clinical ethical disputes during life. Some forum in which relatives can participate is needed, as Gillon [8] pointed out, in addition to ethical guidelines. The Department of Health see this as a matter for local and professional discussion and are unlikely to give guidance. They have however commissioned guidelines on pain management.

I would like to move on to discuss the value of hydration in symptom control, and to consider the problem of thirst.

Fainsinger and colleagues on the palliative care unit in Edmonton Alberta, now offer subcutaneous fluids to all their patients who are dehydrated or likely to become so, because dehydration can cause unpleasant symptoms. They find that about two thirds of their patients, especially those who deteriorate slowly, need subcutaneous fluids, and they are given for 14 days on average.[9]

The consequences and symptoms of dehydration are summarised in Table 1, which is based largely on information from Fainsinger et. al. with some additions of my own. As you see dehydration can cause confusion and restlessness, a dry mouth, impaired speech, thirst, an increased risk of bed sores, circulatory failure and renal failure. Renal failure causes hyperkalaemia and cardiac arrest. A rise in morphine metabolites may cause additional symptoms as indicated. The end result of dehydration is death.

Table 1: The consequence and symptoms of dehydration

Confusion and restlessness*
Dry mouth*
Impaired speech
Thirst*
Increased risk of bed sores*
Circulatory failure
Renal failure*, hyperkalaemia, cardiac arrest
Rise in opioid metabolites* confusion, constipation, nausea,
                                        myoclonus, seizures*
Death

*After Fainsinger et al 1994

Given the ease with which dehydration can be prevented, it is neither kind nor necessary to leave it untreated.

The problem of thirst is of great concern. McCann and co-workers found thirst or a dry mouth to be a major symptom in 66% of patients,. but it tended to decrease as death approached.[10] It has been suggested that cancer patients have a reduced thirst sensation. This is an interesting possibility, but how good I wonder is the evidence? Those who think only in terms of symptom control will argue that if thirst is reduced, dehydration is irrelevant and fluids unnecessary. I would argue that if thirst is reduced, patients are at increased risk of dehydration, as Phillip's group have shown in the healthy elderly.[11] Neglect of dehydration could lead to an escalating spiral of decline. Attention to hydration could improve the prognosis.

There is scope for important research here, to determine whether thirst really is reduced, and if so, what is the mechanism? Could it be for example, due to drugs, to tumour cytokines, or to destruction of nerve pathways by tumour? According to McCullagh, unless the hypothalamic thirst centre is destroyed, thirst can persist even in the presence of severe damage to other parts of the brain.'[2] In the absence of firm evidence it is not safe to assume that dehydrated terminally ill patients do not suffer from thirst.

Traditional methods of suppressing thirst by moistening the mouth may give only transient relief. Physiologists report that thirst quenching involves three phases that are sequential and overlapping, as shown in Figure 1. This is taken from a chapter by Verbalis in a book on thirst, published by Springer-Verlag in 1991.[13] As you see there is an initial oro-pharyngeal phase involving neural reflexes that are provoked by the act of swallowing liquids. This is followed by a gastrointestinal phase due to gastric distension by fluid, and

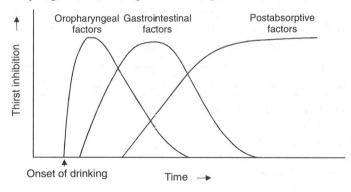

Figure 1: Schematic diagram depicting the onset and duration of various inhibitory signals to continued fluid ingestion following initiation of drinking in response to body fluid deficits. Although each signal by itself is capable of terminating ingestion (depending upon the species), it is the overlapping nature of these sequentially activated mechanisms that produces and sustains the inhibition of further water ingestion. (From Verbalis (1991), with permission.)

finally there is a postabsorptive phase as the fluid restores plasma osmolality to normal. Therefore sustained thirst relief is best achieved with fluid replacement. To try to suppress thirst without giving fluids makes little physiological sense.

Fluid balance is closely monitored and delicately controlled by the body. Figure 2, from the work of Robertson shows the relationship of thirst and plasma vasopressin to plasma solute concentration, or osmolality.[14] As you see, with rising plasma osmolality there is a rise in the hormone vasopressin and a rise in thirst levels. The resulting increase in drinking and in renal fluid retention restores the situation to normal in health. Vasopressin and thirst are controlled by similar monitoring systems, and vasopressin is thought to enhance osmotic thirst.

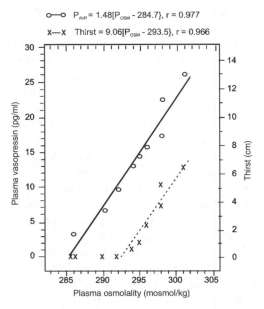

o—o $P_{AVP} = 1.48[P_{OSM} - 284.7]$, r = 0.977

x---x Thirst = $9.06[P_{OSM} - 293.5]$, r = 0.966

Figure 2: The relationship of thirst and plasma vasopressin to plasma osmolality during the infusion of hypertonic saline in a healthy adult. Thirst values are expressed in centimetres from the starting point of an analogue rating scale. (From Robertson (1984), with permission.)

Central release of vasopressin is influenced by endorphins[15] and prostaglandins amongst other things, so morphine and other drugs may impair fluid balance control, and alter thirst unpredictably. It is best to consider all patients on morphine and sedatives to be at risk of dehydration. The greater the level of sedation, the greater the risk. Even lightly sedated patients, especially the elderly, may drink too little and become quietly dehydrated, unnoticed in a corner of the room. Heavily sedated patients on midazolam for example, will be unable to drink at all. If hydration is withheld prolonged dehydration will end in death, whatever the pathology. Even a fit Bedu tribesman, riding in the desert at night can survive for only seven days without food or water. What chance therefore do patients have?

Finally a word about the legal dangers of withholding hydration in terminal care. This is an area of great difficulty on which few lawyers are prepared to express an opinion. However it is quite clear that to sedate a patient and deliberately withhold hydration until the patient dies, leaves the medical team on very shaky legal ground. Mr Justice Ognall, speaking at the Medico-Legal Society pointed out that the distinction between deliberate acts intended to kill, and letting die, is not free from difficulties. He said 'Is a doctor who allows a terminally ill patient to die guilty of murder? Our law says *no,* but providing his intention in omitting to act is to hasten the patient's death, what is the distinction in that circumstance, between an act on the one hand, and an omission on the other?' [16] That I think is the key question. Some lawyers are now saying that a law is needed to prohibit intentional killing by omission.

The law as it stands is generous to the medical profession, and it is open to abuse. It is not morally justifiable to invoke the doctrine of double effect in a doctor's defence, if the doctor has, by intent or oversight, failed to treat predictable and potentially lethal side effects of medication, such as dehydration. [17,18] Doctors are legally responsible for their acts and their omissions.

Sadly there are times when sedation without hydration seems tantamount to euthanasia. This is bad for the image of the hospice movement and strengthens the hand of those who are pressing to legalise physician-assisted suicide. Good palliative medicine is a major defence against euthanasia, but please heed my warning. Sedation without hydration has enormous potential for misuse. I would like to see this regime consigned to the dustbin of history. If you look at what is happening in Northern Australia you will see the dangers clearly. Their self-deliverance homicide machine mark 2 induces coma—you may be sure that it does not hydrate! Closer to home a doctor, speaking in London, told how a man with advanced motor neurone disease had asked to be killed. 'I can't do that' replied the doctor, 'but I can make you unaware of your situation'. So he sedated the man and withheld hydration until he died. 'What was I supposed to say?' he asked when challenged— 'Tell him that I could do nothing? A doctor's duty is to relieve suffering.'

In the case of Annie Lindsell, who sought euthanasia, her doctor was careful to state that he intended to sedate her when her motor neurone disease affected her swallowing. The High Court case was withdrawn without a judicial ruling. [19] The Judge warned that he could not grant Ms Lindsell's doctor immunity from prosecution.

Ultimately what is on trial in all this is the integrity of the medical and legal professions. The doctrine of double effect must not be used as a smoke screen for euthanasia.

The main dangers of withholding hydration that I have touched on are shown in Table 2.

Table 2: Main dangers of withholding hydration
Dehydration and death
Ethical and legal problems
Abuse of power by doctors
Thirst and other symptoms
Hell for relatives

I have said enough about the death-orientated approach. I will end by considering a life-orientated, life-supportive approach to palliative care. This is summarised in Table 3. As you see many of the features tally with the best traditions of the hospice movement. Doctors with this approach will support life in comfort and dignity, do no harm, attend to the mental, spiritual and physical needs of the patient, and will be sensitive to relatives. They will treat symptoms safely and use technology wisely, not only for pain relief, but also to maintain hydration, if possible to the end, providing that fluid administration is not in itself a burden to the patient. Application of this ethical principle, put forward by the House of Lord's Select Committee on Medical Ethics, would simplify many difficult treatment limiting decisions.

Table 3: Life oriented approach to terminal care
Support life in comfort and dignity.
Do no harm.
Attend to mental, spiritual and physical needs.
Be sensitive to relatives.
Treat symptoms safely.
Use technology wisely.
Maintain hydration if possible to the end.

The message I would like you to take home with you is that *'Attention to hydration is not merely optional, it should be a basic part of good medicine and good palliative care.'*

Finally there is a wider aspect to this debate that takes us beyond the realm of science and medicine, into the realm of the human heart and spirit. Human life is precious, we do not pass this way again. We as doctors, have a special duty to support life wisely, until it comes to a natural end. It is not our role to launch the soul on it's longest journey. Heaven can wait.

Acknowledgements

This paper was based on one given by Gilllian Craig at a conference on palliative care in general medicine, at the Royal College of Physicians of London on June 4th 1997.[20] For a fuller discussion of ethical and legal aspects readers are referred elsewhere. [1, 16-18]

Addendum. A relative's testimony

A member of the public commented "I would like to confirm what Dr Craig has said... My husband had cancer and suffered pain in his left leg. He went to a hospice for pain control. He was, and remained, clear in his mind and showed no sign of immediate terminal illness. We thought we had a lot more living to do together.

"One night, without consultation, a doctor made the decision and changed my husband's medication. I learnt later that he was being given midazolam. My request for him to receive sustenance was ignored, he drifted into a coma and died seven days later. His tongue was so dehydrated it had curled up tight at the back of his throat.

"My Member of Parliament gave every support in trying to get two independent medical opinions, which I feel I am entitled to, but to no avail. It seems to me that the National Health Service complaints procedure is failing the ordinary person in the street. Most of us cannot afford legal advice.

"I have never been able to grieve. My whole existence has been affected by the way my husband died. What ever deliberations are made in the future, the public must be protected."

Source confidential. Quoted with permission.

References

1. Craig, G.M., 'On withholding nutrition and hydration in the terminally ill: has palliative medicine gone too far?' *Journal of Medical Ethics* 1994;**20:** 139-143.

2. Artifical hydration (AH) for people who are terminally ill. *European Journal of Palliative Care* 1997;**4:** 124. See also *ibid.* pp. 26-128 for the background to the guidelines.

3. Neale I., 'A basic lesson relearnt. The singing histopathologist', *British Medical Journal* 1997;**314**: 333.

4. Cameron H.M. and McGoogan E., 'A prospective study of 1152 hospital autopsies: Inaccuracies in death certification', *Journal of Pathology* 1981;**133**: 273-283.

5. The autopsy and audit. Report of the Joint Working Party of the Royal College of Pathologists, the Royal College of Physicians of London, and the Royal College of Surgeons of England, 1991.

6. Blake W., 'The Garden of Love' in *The London Book of English Verse,* (London: Eyre and Spottiswoode), p.292.

7. Report of the committee of inquiry into South Ockendon Hospital. Para 533 p. 137, HMSO 1974.

8. Gillon R., 'Palliative care ethics: non-provision of artificial nutrition and hydration to terminally ill sedated patients', *Journal of Medical Ethics* 1994;**20**: 131-132, 187.

9. Fainsinger R.L., MacEarchern T., Miller M.J. et. al., 'The use of hypodermoclysis for rehydration in terminally ill cancer patients', *Journal of Pain and Symptom Management* 1994;**9**: 298-302.
10. McCann R.M., Hall W.J., Groth-Juncker A., 'Comfort care for terminally ill patients. The appropriate use of nutrition and hydration', *Journal of the American Medical Association* 1994;**272**: 1263-1266.
11. Phillips P., Rolls B.J., Ledingham J.G.G. et al., 'Reduced thirst after water deprivation in healthy elderly men', *New England Journal of Medicine* 1984;**311**: 753-9.
12. McCullagh P., 'Thirst in relation to withdrawal of hydration', *Catholic Medical Quarterly* 1996;XL,VI: 5-12.
13. Verbalis J.G., Fig. 19.5 in *Thirst: Physiological and Psychological Aspects.* Ed Ramsay D.J. and Booth DA. Springer-Verlag, (London 1991), p.325 Used with permission.
14. Robertson G., 'Abnormalities of thirst regulation (nephrology forum)', *Kidney International* 25, Figure 2 page 462, 1984. Copyright International Society of Nephrology. Used with permission.
15. Lightman S.L. and Forsling ML., 'Evidence for endogenous opioid control of vasopressin release in man', *Journal of Clinical Endocrinology and Metabolism.* 1980; **50**: 569-571.
16. Ognall H., 'A right to die? Some medico-legal reflection', *Medico-legal Journal* 1994;**4**: 165-179.
17. Craig G.M., 'Is sedation without hydration or nourishment in terminal care lawful?', *Medico-legal Journal* 1994;**4:** 198-201.
18. Craig G.M., 'On withholding artificial hydration and nutrition from terminally ill sedated patients. The debate continues', *Journal of Medical Ethics* 1996;**22:** 147-153.
19. Dyer C., 'Court confirms right to palliative treatment for mental distress', *British Medical Journal* 1997;**315**: 1178.
20. Conference reports, 'Palliative care in general medicine', *Journal of the Royal College of Physicians of London* 1997;**31**: 695-69.

Chapter 8

Some Areas of Concern

1. Death from dehydration: Some pros and cons

Author Gillian Craig

Given the fact that water is essential for life, many observers find it deeply distressing to see a person deprived of fluids and unable to drink at the end of life. Relatives who have seen their loved ones die in this way may be comforted to know that some people think it is not too bad a way to die. Some even advocate it as an alternative to doctor-assisted suicide for those who seek an exit from life.[1]

Most people who are deprived of fluids will die within a week or two. Occasional cases are reported in the literature where patients survived for several weeks without fluids. This could only be explained on the basis of gross fluid overload at the outset of fluid deprivation. Clinical judgement and common sense must be used when interpreting such reports.

If a comfortable and peaceful death is your aim for a patient who is dying, dehydration has long been regarded as satisfactory, provided that attempts are made to assuage thirst by moistening the mouth. I am somewhat sceptical about this approach to the problem of thirst for reasons that I outlined earlier. It does not make much physiological sense. Nevertheless, some would argue that maintaining physiological equilibrium is only necessary if it is of benefit to the patient. If remaining alive is not regarded as a benefit, some would say that physiological equilibrium is of little consequence.

Advocates of 'managed death' point to several advantages for dehydration as a mode of death. It is they say "natural", it requires no outside help, it provides "a comfortable exit from life", and it will ensure that dying will not be unduly protracted.[1] Palliative care specialists see additional advantages, some of which are mentioned elsewhere in this book. They argue that reduced urine output makes nursing easier, they claim that thirst is not a problem in cancer patients and argue that giving fluids does not prevent thirst. They suggest that dehydration reduces respiratory secretions, and they magnify the problems of drips. They even suggest that dehydration can be helpful in certain types of pain. There may be a grain of truth in some of these comments but they need closer examination.

1. The question of thirst

There is at present very little hard evidence that thirst is reduced in patients dying of cancer, but it is theoretically possible, for reasons that I discussed earlier. It is certainly a comforting thought that nature in its wisdom may have found a way to reduce distress when people no longer have the strength to drink. For a multitude of reasons it is difficult to get hard research evidence in the dying. Undeterred, some palliative carers simply point out that "an absence of evidence does not mean that a service or treatment is not effective, simply that we do not know".[2]

There is some evidence to suggest that thirst is reduced to some extent in elderly people, even apparently healthy elderly people.[3] This may be an indication of changes in central nerve responses – a gradual running down due to age. There is also some evidence that thirst is reduced in people suffering from multiple system atrophy [4] - a condition rather similar to Alzheimer's disease.

There are theoretical grounds for believing that thirst may be reduced under many different circumstances in sick people. The clues can be found in work done largely on animals and the evidence is available in textbooks.[5] Possible mechanisms for thirst reduction are listed in Table 1.

Table 1 Possible mechanisms for thirst reduction in sick people [5]
Fluid overload
Hypoxia
Changes in vasopressin levels
Reduced angiotensin II levels
Reduced plasma osmolality
Structural damage to receptors
Structural damage to neuroendocrine circuits
Degenerative change in the brain
Medication e.g. nitroprusside, papaverine, ACE inhibitors
Tumour cytokines
Prostaglandins, especially the E series
Tachykinins – substance P and neurokinins
Gastric distension by fluid

The observation that patients dying of cancer often stop drinking as death approaches, does not necessarily mean that they no longer feel thirsty. They may stop drinking because they are too weak to hold a cup, too tired to bother, or no longer able to swallow for one reason or another.

Thus, although thirst may be reduced in some dying patients, it is not safe to assume that dehydrated dying patients do not experience thirst. They are likely to do so unless the thirst centre in the brain has been damaged by disease or is rendered ineffective by circulating hormones, or other factors.

2. Abnormal thirst perception

The observation that giving fluids does not always relieve thirst in the dying, suggests either that insufficient fluid has been given or that there is an abnormality of thirst perception.

If a person who is normally hydrated experiences thirst, the physician should review the patient's medication. Drugs with atropine-like qualities are often used in palliative medicine to reduce respiratory secretions. One of the classical symptoms of atropine overdose is thirst. Many anti-depressant drugs which are used widely in palliative care, have anti-cholinergic properties and can cause a dry mouth which may be misinterpreted as thirst.

Years ago, in the mid 1930s McCance reported that experimental salt deficiency can result in a sensation akin to thirst. One subject noted that he felt "Thirsty all morning – drank a lot, but water seemed to make no difference." Another day he reported a "funny feeling in the mouth". All subjects felt apathetic, anorexic and exhausted. They recovered dramatically on eating salt. A female subject noted that her sense of flavour and taste returned within half-an-hour, although no fluid had been taken. This she spoke of as a quenching of thirst. "Genuine and almost unbearable thirst supervened later and was only satisfied by copious draughts of water", wrote McCance.[6]

Very sick patients often have what is described as 'sick cell syndrome'. Their plasma sodium is low and plasma potassium raised although there may be no overall lack of body sodium. Bearing in mind the work of McCance it seems quite possible that such patients could have some alteration of thirst perception through mechanisms that are as yet not understood. This would add to the difficulties of studying thirst in the dying.

3. Practical considerations

It has been suggested that since the timing of death is fairly predictable when fluids are withdrawn, death from dehydration may have certain practical advantages.[1] This may well be true. Family and friends can cancel engagements and arrange to be present. In contrast, dying from an unpredictable disease process rather than from untreated dehydration, can be an uncertain process. It is astonishing how confident hospice doctors can be about the timing of death - but perhaps it should not be astonishing for they see death from dehydration so often.

Anecdotal evidence suggests that dehydration may be beneficial in pain. A possible mechanism might be that oedema fluid and swelling could be reduced with potential benefit if pain is due to nerve compression. However, the benefit will be short lived, for the patient will die. There are better ways of treating pain! Similarly, reduced urine output may be beneficial in the short term if the patient is incontinent or finds it painful to move, but after a few days of anuria death will occur from kidney failure and a raised serum potassium. So to a life-orientated physician all these arguments in favour of dehydration are specious and unconvincing. To a death-orientated doctor they may carry some weight.

4. Other considerations

Death from dehydration is 'natural' it is claimed.[1] This is true to the extent that it is inevitable if no medical help is at hand and you are unable to drink. If you are in the desert with no water for days you will die of dehydration naturally. If you lived in the days before artificial hydration was invented and you could not swallow, you died of dehydration - naturally. However, in my view it is unnatural and wrong to withhold fluids from dying patients when you have the power to maintain hydration quite simply until the end.

Sometimes dehydration is self-induced. Some people decide of their own accord to stop drinking with a view to ending their life. People who make this decision may be old, depressed, lonely, isolated, ill, confused or reluctant to struggle on with disability. Some can be dissuaded by gentleness and social support. Others continue relentlessly on their course of self-destruction and achieve their aim.

It is extremely distressing to all concerned when people take matters into their own hands in this way. Friends, family and health care professionals are liable to feel hurt and rejected. To express your autonomy in this way can be perceived as a very inconsiderate act. You run the risk of leaving behind a legacy of emotional pain. On the other hand some families might see it as an act of courage and altruism, but I am inclined to think that such families would be few and far between. Most would sadly accept the old person's decision that the time had come to depart.

Some people who fear incapacity, drips and tube feeding may sign their own death warrant in advance, through an advance directive. They may not appreciate that by so doing they run the risk of dying of dehydration quite unnecessarily. Many a person has survived to live a full and active life after a period of temporary incapacity necessitating these life-supportive measures.

If a person is truly terminally ill and actively dying, no doctor on earth can prevent death. Life cannot be prolonged indefinitely under such circumstances even with artificial hydration. The average length of time that patients in a hospice need subcutaneous fluids is 14 days before death occurs from natural causes. Those days could be precious to the patient and their family.

When a person is not actively dying and can be kept alive by artificial hydration and nutrition for weeks, months, or years, the ethical problems posed by withholding artificial hydration or nutrition are rather different. Some would say totally different. It is a very serious matter indeed for a doctor to take a decision to deliberately dehydrate someone who is not terminally ill or dying. Dr Richard Lamerton, an experienced hospice doctor commented - "The debate hinges on whether artificial hydration is medical treatment or not; but is that the point? If it is only nursing treatment does that alter it? Treatment has one of two aims – curing or avoiding distress. By whatever means, providing water is a simple duty to avoid distress. Withdrawing it puts doctors in a new world of value judgements which are very dangerous. Those of my colleagues who are happy to dance across this minefield are the very ones I would be most scared of if I found myself in hospital after a stroke and unable to communicate".[7]

Acknowledgement and note

This paper was first published in the Catholic Medical Quarterly (CMQ) in May 2001. At the same time, at the request of Dr Craig, the Editor also published the National Council for Hospice and Specialist Palliative Care Services guidelines on the ethical use of artificial hydration in terminally ill patients as it was felt that they had not received sufficient publicity.

References

1   Hoefler J M. The dehydration alternative. p.117-123. In Managing Death. *Westview Press* 1997.
2   Higginson I J. Evidence based palliative care. *British Medical Journal*. 1999; **319**: 462-3.
3   Phillips P, Rolls B J, Ledingham J G G. *et al*. Reduced thirst after water deprivation in health elderly men. *New England Journal of Medicine*. 1994; **311**: 753-9.

4   Bevilacqua M, Norbiato G, Righini V. *et al.* Loss of   osmotic thirst in multiple system atrophy: association with sinoaortic baroreceptor deafferentation. *American Journal of Physiology*. 1994; **266**: 1752-8.

5   Thirst. Physiological and Psychological Aspects. (Eds.) Ramsay D J and Booth D A. *Springer-Verlag*. London. 1991.

6   McCance R A. Experimental sodium chloride deficiency in man. Proceedings of the Royal Society of London. Series B. Biological Sciences **119**, 245-268. 1935-1936.

7   Lamerton R. Comments on BMA guidance, from a statement sent to MPs in January 2000.

A response from Dame Cicely Saunders

The above article provoked a strong response from Dame Cicely Saunders, in her role as Founder and President of the National Council for Hospice and Specialist Palliative Care Services (NCHSPCS). Dame Cicely wrote to Dr Peter Doherty, Editor of the Catholic Medical Quarterly. Her letter was published in the Catholic Medical Quarterly of August 2001 (p21) as follows:-

'I am very glad that the paper from The National Council for Hospice and Specialist Palliative Care Services on Ethical Decision Making in Palliative Care followed the paper from Dr Gillian Craig – Death from Dehydration – some pros and cons (CMQ May 2001.)

'I would like to point out that contrary to Dr Craig's comment in that article, hospice doctors do not see death from dehydration 'often'. In fact, at St Christopher's, we have used subcutaneous hydration for some 70 patients (out of a total of 1600) and would always respond in this way if necessary.

'Patients do not die from dehydration – they die from the disease. It is important your readers know this.'

Dr Craig replied as follows in a letter to the Editor of the CMQ:-

'May I respond to correspondence generated by my recent article 'Death from dehydration – some pros and cons' (CMQ May 2001)? It is difficult to continue an important debate when some people deny that there is a problem. Dame Cicely Saunders takes issue with my comment that hospice doctors see dehydration 'often', and quotes figures indicating that some 4.3% of patients at St Christopher's Hospice receive subcutaneous (SC) fluids, when 'necessary'. (CMQ August 2001).

'This low figure proves my point, for Fainsinger et. al. have shown that when sc fluids are offered to all hospice patients who are dehydrated, or at risk of becoming so, the uptake is 69%.(i) The disparity suggests that many patients who might benefit from hydration are not given sc fluids at St Christopher's. It all depends on whether sc fluids are considered "necessary". Those who follow the traditional "comfort care only" philosophy have one view, those who treat dehydration in order to support life see things rather differently. McCann et al, writing from a hospital perspective in 1994, admitted that 'It is probable that most of our patients die with dehydration.' (ii).

'The situation has improved a little in the UK, thanks to the efforts of the palliative carers but there is still some way to go. The NCHSPCS guidelines are helpful but have not received the publicity they deserved and tend to be overlooked by those who should know better. Some palliative carers still argue that dehydration in advanced illness 'does not seem to cause physical discomfort and need not be treated.'(iii). In short a somewhat Luddite approach to hydration prevails, with the full support of economists and utilitarian philosophers. Death from dehydration remains a very real danger, even in the best regulated circles.

References

(i) Fainsinger R.L. et al. *Journal of Pain and Symptom Management.* 1994; **9**: 298-392.
(ii) McCann R.M. et al. *Journal of the American Medical Association.* 1994; **272**: 1263-6.
(iii) Billings J.A. *British Medical Journal.* 2000; **321**: 555-8.

2. Terminal sedation

Author Gillian Craig.

Abstract

This paper highlights the dangers of terminal sedation – a controversial aspect of palliative care. The author drew attention to the dangers of sedation without hydration some years ago (Journal of Medical Ethics 1994; 20:139-143) and debated the issues at the Royal College of Physicians in 1997 (Ethics & Medicine 1999; 15.1:15-19).

The author shows how advocates of euthanasia in the UK and elsewhere are exploiting the practice of "terminal sedation" and considers their allegations. The ethical and legal risks of sedation would be greatly reduced if palliative carers took a more active approach to hydration.

Sedation when given with the sole intention of relieving suffering at the end of life has become an accepted but highly controversial aspect of palliative care. Some years ago I warned that the practice of sedation without hydration would strengthen the hand of those who sought to promote euthanasia. My warning proved true! Advocates of euthanasia on both sides of the Atlantic are now trying to exploit the practice of 'terminal sedation' or 'slow euthanasia' for their own ends. Take for example an article by Irwin in the Voluntary Euthanasia News of May 2001.[1]

Dr Michael Irwin is a prominent member of the Voluntary Euthanasia Society in the UK and acts as their main spokesman. He attended the biennial conference of the World Federation of Right-To-Die Societies that was held in the USA in September 2000. According to Irwin, 70 participating doctors signed the 'Boston Declaration on Assisted Dying', the main paragraph of which states:

"We wish to draw public attention to the practice of 'terminal sedation' or 'slow euthanasia' which is performed extensively today throughout the world in hospitals, nursing homes, hospices and in private homes …. a physician may lawfully administer increasing dosages of regular analgesic and sedative drugs that can hasten someone's death as long as the declared intention is to ease pain and suffering …. Compassionate physicians, without publicly declaring the true intention of their actions, often speed up the dying process in this way. Many thousands of terminally-ill patients are so helped globally every year." [1]

Reporting back to members in the UK, Irwin wrote: "For VES members, I believe it is important that we stress that terminal sedation, both voluntary and involuntary … is widely performed in this country, especially in hospices and nursing homes, and as it is totally uncontrolled, this procedure is open to abuse." [1]

The allegations in the Boston declaration are serious, but difficult to substantiate. When a patient is dying it is hard to prove beyond all reasonable doubt that life was shortened by the treatment given. Nevertheless concerns about "slow euthanasia", a term used by Billings and Block in 1996 [2], have focussed minds and stimulated research considerably in recent years. However, as the Tumim Committee observed in their position statement in March 2001, "While there is a widespread belief that voluntary euthanasia occurs in the UK, its prevalence is a matter for conjecture… The procedure's illegality makes reliable information impossible to obtain." [3]

In recent years serious attempts have been made to gather hard information about the use of sedation in terminally ill patients. However very few people have attempted to study the relationship between sedation and dehydration. In a highly controversial paper written in 1997, Quill and colleagues considered "palliative options of last resort", and compared voluntarily stopping eating and drinking, terminal sedation, physician-assisted suicide and voluntary active euthanasia. They argued that "Terminal sedation and voluntarily stopping eating and drinking would allow clinicians to remain responsive to a wide range of patient suffering, but they are ethically and clinically more complex, and closer to physician-assisted suicide and voluntary active euthanasia than is ordinarily acknowledged." Various safeguards were proposed for any medical action that may hasten death.[4] Their paper provoked much critical comment from people who considered the proposals immoral and unethical.[5]

Published estimates of the number of patients requiring sedation for intractable symptoms at the end of life vary widely. Initial reports by Ventafridda gave a high incidence of sedation in the region of 52% [6]. Fainsinger and colleagues in a multicentre international study found that the "intent to sedate" in hospices in Israel, Durban, Cape Town and Madrid varied from 15% to 36%, sedation being defined as when the patient was made unresponsive in order to achieve comfort. Sedation with midazolam was used in most cases. Wide cultural variations were found, particularly with respect to sedation for delirium; the use of sedation for this symptom varying from 15% in Durban to 60% in Madrid. The use of sedation for other symptoms showed less marked variations between centres. In general about 80% of the patients studied needed medical management for pain, 40% for nausea and vomiting, and 25 to 53% for shortness of breath. The authors commented "We need to be mindful of the suggestion that with careful assessment of reversible factors and alternative management for problems like delirium, some of the need for sedation may be avoided." [7]

Within nations individual physicians are likely to have different thresholds for intervention. Treatment may also be influenced by factors such as the stoicism and wishes of the patient. Some patients, for example if given a choice, may prefer to avoid sedation, whereas others who fear impending disability and death, may request sedation at a relatively early stage in their illness. As Irwin notes "The very wide variations in the frequency of sedation among different medical centres suggest that the choice to sedate patients may reflect doctor's behaviour or the organisation's policies rather than the patient's preferences or needs." [1] I am reminded of Main's observation about the risk of inappropriate sedation! However, very often some degree of sedation, chosen with skill and sensitivity is essential for the patient's comfort.

Thorns and Sykes, reporting a retrospective study of the use of opioids in the last week of life in 238 consecutive hospice patients concluded that "appropriate use of opioids does not shorten life and there is little if any need to invoke DDE." (DDE is short for doctrine of double effect.) 28 of their patients had a marked increase in opioids in the last week of life, mainly for pain, shortness of breath or cough, and all were on some unspecified sedation. No comment was made about the use or otherwise of hydration. The authors found no significant difference in survival between patients who had a marked increase in opioids in the last week of life, and those who did not. They comment "The DDE may be a useful principle that can offer reassurance to health-care professionals facing difficult treatment decisions, but it must be distinguished from euthanasia and its role should not be exaggerated." [8]

Published reports tend to confirm the view that sedation is widely used at the end of life, but the link between sedation and death has not been established. Delegates at the Right-to-Die Conference in Boston were undaunted by such difficulties. Perhaps they had access to inside information about their own activities. Perhaps it suited their purposes to exaggerate the situation. On the other hand, perhaps they were indeed telling the truth, for there is no smoke without fire! What is needed now is some good research to determine whether sedated patients who are hydrated survive longer than sedated patients who are left without hydration. Common sense suggests that they will.

Irwin argues that the practice of terminal sedation amounts to euthanasia "because the comatose patient often dies from the combination of two intentional acts by a doctor – the induction of unconsciousness, and the withholding of food and water …. And so, for many, terminal sedation is really Society's wink to euthanasia, for on the surface it looks like a combination of the accepted practices of aggressive comfort care and the withdrawal of life-sustaining treatment." Irwin sees the practice of terminal sedation "as a form of psychological defence mechanism for palliative care practitioners, allowing them to focus on keeping a terminally ill patient in a pharmacological oblivion rather than acknowledge that they may be actively ending someone's life." [1]

At the Right-to-Die meeting in Boston, several American physicians were reported to be "concerned that the palliative care movement, especially in the United States, was generally encouraging terminal sedation as a 'good medical practice' which could eventually be seen as a better alternative to physician-assisted suicide or voluntary euthanasia." [1] Irwin concedes that by "creating the illusion of a natural death and avoiding the sense of urgency for some terminally ill patients and their families, slow euthanasia may be more acceptable than rapid and fully acknowledged euthanasia." This worries advocates of the lethal injection approach who are campaigning for the right to die by "rapidly effective lethal drugs." However, they hope to sway public opinion in this direction by various ploys. They will no doubt emphasise the disadvantages of "slow euthanasia", referring to this as a lingering death, with loss of dignity and distortion of the memory left in the minds of loved ones, in the hope that the public will clamour for a quick exit.[1] These points may be valid in some cases, but in general the public should be wary of propaganda and the use of emotive language. A lingering death for example, may also be a peaceful death that allows loved ones time to accept the inevitable. A calm but sedated person, lovingly cared for, need not lack dignity. Take away the propaganda factor and many of the points raised by advocates of euthanasia carry little weight.

I do however share the view that prolonged sedation without hydration is, on occasions, tantamount to euthanasia. I also feel that the hospice movement has not fully grasped the nettle of dehydration, nor fully addressed the implications of their reluctance to maintain hydration at the end of life. I hope that the forceful views of the Right-to-Die movement will encourage palliative carers to take a more active approach to hydration. In my view the legal and ethical problems of terminal sedation could be overcome quite simply by providing hydration for a matter of days until life ends naturally. The provision of life supportive fluids is surely preferable to death by lethal injection.

No one should underestimate the difficulties that palliative care workers face. Their main aim is to ensure that dying patients do not suffer. Most workers in the specialty are, to quote a leading article in the Lancet "ardently opposed to any form of euthanasia ..." [9]

However, it must also be recognised that some people working in the field see things rather differently. Take for example the aforementioned article by Quill [4] or a disturbing review by Billings who advocates the practice of sedation without hydration for the relief of intractable suffering in the dying patient.[10]

Current legislation protects doctors whose intentions are honourable. Intentional killing by a deliberate act remains unlawful in the UK and in most other countries at present. However doctors remain extremely sensitive to close scrutiny of their actions at the end of life and are wary of any legislation that might limit their clinical freedom.[11] Doctors whose primary aim is to control pain and distress are well protected by current legislation. Nevertheless concerns expressed by sections of the medical profession in recent years have helped to block broader anti-euthanasia legislation in the UK and in the USA. I refer to the Medical Treatment (Prevention of Euthanasia) Bill in the UK and the Pain Relief Promotion Act in the USA. One can only hope that new legislation will be devised that will prevent euthanasia by act or omission, while enabling doctors with honourable intentions, to control pain and other distressing symptoms at the end of life.

According to Hardy there is now concern "that sedation as the best means of symptom control in the dying patient may be underused because of the fear of employing "terminal sedation" [9] – in other words, because of concerns about euthanasia. Rather similar concerns are raised from time to time about the use of opioids, for it is alleged that fear of prosecution may prevent doctors from prescribing adequate doses for pain relief.[11] However, in skilled hands, opioids do not shorten life. Equally, in skilled hands, and with careful attention to hydration, sedation need not and should not shorten life.

Acknowledgement

This paper was first published in the Catholic Medical Quarterly in February 2002.

References

1   Irwin M. Terminal sedation. Voluntary Euthanasia News. May 2001 p8-9.

2   Billings JA. Block SD. Slow euthanasia. *Journal of Palliative Care*. 1996; **12**: 21-30.

3   Medical treatment at the end of life. A position statement. *Clinical Medicine* 2001;**1**: 116.

4   Quill TW. Lo B. Brock DW. Palliative options of last resort: a comparison of stopping eating and drinking, terminal sedation, physician-assisted suicide, and voluntary active euthanasia. *Journal of the American Medical Association*. 1997; **278**: 2099-2104.

5   Letters. Howsepian A. and others. *Journal of the American Medical Association*. 1998; **279**: 1066-7.

6   Ventafridda V. Ripamonti C. deConno F. et al. Symptom prevalence and control during cancer patients' last days of life. *Journal of Palliative Care*. 1990; **6**:7-11.

7   Fainsinger RL. Waller A. Bercovici M et al. A multicentre international study of sedation for uncontrolled symptoms in terminally ill patients. *Palliative Medicine*. 2000; **14**: 257-65.

8   Thorns A. Sykes N. Opioid use in last week of life and implications for end-of-life decision making. *The Lancet*. 2000; **356**: 398-9.

9   Hardy J. Sedation in terminally ill patients. *The Lancet*. 2000; **356**: 1866-7.

10 Billings JA. Recent advances in palliative care. *British Medical Journal*. 2000; **321**: 555-558.

11 Baumrucker SJ. Should we fear the Pain Relief Promotion Act? *American Journal of Hospice and Palliative Care*. 2000; **17**: 224-226.

3. Sedated to death?

When "comfort care" becomes dangerous.

Author Nancy Guilfoy Valko, RN.

As I write this in May 2002, the Haiwaiian legislature has just defeated a bill to legalise assisted suicide by only three votes. Few people were aware of how close Hawaii came to joining Oregon as the second US state to allow doctors to help kill their patients. But before anyone breathes a sigh of relief, it is important to understand that a quieter - but just as lethal - advance in the euthanasia agenda is gaining ground in the US.

In the past few years, some ethicists and doctors have proposed "terminal sedation" (TS) as a legal alternative to assisted suicide. TS is defined as the deliberate "termination of awareness" for "relief of intractable pain when specific pain relieving protocols or interventions are ineffective" and/or "relief of intractable *emotional or spiritual anguish* (existential suffering, psychological distress, emotional exhaustion)". (Emphasis added). An essential component of TS is also the withdrawal of treatment, including even food and water, so that death occurs as soon as possible.

The issue is not really "intractable pain", which those of us who have worked in a hospice or with dying patients know can virtually always be controlled. In Oregon, voters were sold the assisted suicide law by claims that terminally ill people needed lethal overdoses to relieve unbearable pain- yet even the limited data on assisted suicide victims there shows that the main reasons given by the victims were fear of future suffering, losing independence and/or being a "burden" on family members rather than current or unbearable pain.

While some euthanasia supporters have called TS "inhumane" compared with the faster death by lethal overdose, other supporters view TS as a way of getting around the "problem" of the euthanasia movement's inability, so far to convince voters or state legislatures to enact Oregon-style assisted suicide laws. Increasingly, TS is being incorporated into some hospice and other "end-of-life" programmes, even though, as writer Brian Johnston points out, euthanasia supporters like Doctor David Orentlicher are admitting in prestigious medical journals that "terminal sedation is tantamount to euthanasia, or a kind of slow euthanasia".

Unfortunately, even some doctors who condemn assisted suicide have embraced TS as an ethical "choice". Doctor Ira Brock, a public opponent of assisted suicide, recently joined with Doctor Timothy Quill, an even more public supporter of assisted suicide, in writing an article supporting TS. As an example of the ethical use of TS, they used the case of a radiology doctor with a lethal brain tumour who wanted to die as soon as possible, not because he was in pain but because he was losing his ability to function independently. The radiologist decided to stop all his medications (as well as eating and drinking) but insisted that his doctor make the process bearable.

This demand resulted in the use of TS to alleviate his confusion and agitation, which resulted after nine days without food or water.

Similarly, Dr Robert Kingsbury, the director of SSM (Sisters of Saint Mary) Catholic hospice in St Louis, wrote an article supporting the option of TS as comforting and "critical for patients who are profoundly fearful" of terrible suffering at the end of life. Although the traditional and trusted hospice philosophy has been to care for the dying without either prolonging or hastening death, Doctor Kingsbury rejects the notion that TS and withdrawal of food and water causes or hastens death.

Tellingly, The Pontifical Council's 1994 Charter for Health Care Workers makes an important point when it warns that:

'Sometimes the systematic use of narcotics, which reduce the consciousness of the patient, is a cloak for the frequently unconscious wish of the health care worker to discontinue relating to the dying person. In this case it is not so much the alleviation of the patient's suffering that is sought as the convenience of those in attendance. The dying person is deprived of the possibility of 'living his own life', by reducing him to a state of unconsciousness unworthy of a human being. This is why the administration of narcotics for the sole purpose of depriving the dying person of a conscious end is 'a truly deplorable practice.'

Non-voluntary Terminal Sedation

Although TS is usually presented as an ethical "choice" rationally made by people who are dying, TS is not uncommon even for people who are incompetent to make their own decisions or who are not close to death.

Dr Perry Fine provided the rationale for the use of TS by citing "living wills" and other advance directives, as well as decisions made by family and others. Virtually every "living will" or other advance directive specifically requests medication if needed for pain even if there is a risk of hastening death. While no one would disagree with this principle, the reality is that such language can provide a loophole for doctors or families who see death as something to get over with as soon as possible. Families often agree to "comfort care only" for relatives with brain injuries or dementia without realizing that this can also involve TS.

For example, a few years ago I received a phone call from a niece who was worried about her elderly aunt who had suffered a severe stroke several days before. The aunt had signed a protective document designed by a pro-life group as an alternative to the dangerous "living will". The document specifically said that, unless death was inevitable and imminent, ordinary treatments such as food, water and basic medical care were to be provided. The document also named the aunt's sister as the person to make medical decisions if the aunt became incapacitated.

The problem was that although the doctor had declared the aunt's stroke a "terminal event" (a questionable prognosis at best), she was still alive and breathing, although unconscious. Understandably, the niece began to question whether her aunt was indeed terminal and whether she should be receiving food, water and basic medical care as her protective document directed.

One of the first questions I asked was whether the aunt was on morphine. (Although strokes rarely cause pain beyond a sometimes initial headache, many doctors and nurses consider unconsciousness as a sign that the patient will be severely disabled even if he or she lives, and thus deem such a patient "hopeless".) The niece said that the doctor had ordered the morphine as part of the "comfort care" to prevent any discomfort as the aunt died. I suggested that the niece talk to the doctor and her aunt's sister about stopping or reducing the morphine to see if this was responsible for the aunt's apparent coma. Sure enough, when the morphine was stopped, the aunt began to respond and according to the niece, even seemed to recognize relatives.

However, the aunt's sister insisted that a priest told her such apparent reactions were "just reflexes" and told the doctor to resume the morphine. The other relatives briefly considered talking to a lawyer about enforcing the protective document but were reluctant to cause further division in the family. Not surprisingly the aunt died after two weeks without food and water.

Such scenarios are unfortunately becoming more and more frequent. Terminal sedation is *not* a rarely used last resort, as its supporters maintain. Even the few studies on TS report the prevalence of terminal sedation to range from 3% to 52% in the terminally ill. When the unknown actual incidence of terminating awareness- or ensuring unawareness- in patients with stroke, dementia or other serious illnesses is factored in, the use of TS as a form of "comfort care" may well be approaching epidemic proportions, even outside the hospice area.

As a former hospice nurse and now as an ICU (intensive care unit) nurse caring for some patients who turn out to be dying, I support the appropriate use of pain and sedating medications as ethical comfort care. However, even in circumstances where such medications are necessary, I have never seen a case where a patient "needed" to be made permanently unconscious.

In addition, the newer health care system problems of cost-containment and stressed, overburdened caregivers can make TS even more attractive - and dangerous - to patients, families and medical professionals alike.

The euthanasia movement is nothing if not creative and persistent. Many people now mistakenly believe that tolerating just a little bit of deliberate death- with safeguards, of course- will give them control at the end of their own lives. But as the "culture of death" keeps seducing even well-meaning patients, families and medical professionals into making death decisions based on fear of suffering or diminished quality of life rather than following traditional principles of not causing or hastening death, ultimately we are all at risk of being "compassionately" rationalized to death.

Sources

1. Perry Fine, MD, "Total Sedation in End-of Life Care; Clinical Considerations", *Journal of Hospice and Palliative Care Nursing*, 2001, Vol 3, No 3.
2. Timothy E. Quill, MD and Ira R Brock, MD for the ACP-ASIM End-of-Life Care Consensus Panel, "Responding to Intractable Terminal Suffering: The Role of Terminal Sedation and Voluntary Refusal of Food and Fluids", *Annals of Internal Medicine* 2000; **132**: 408-414. Online version available at http://www.worldrtd.org/quill&Bytock.html

3. Charter for Health Care Workers. *Pontifical Council for Pastoral Assistance.* Vatican translation. 1994; Number 124; p 108. Available online at: http://www.ewtn.com/library/CURIA/PCPAHEAL.HTM.
4. Tina Maluso-Bolton, MN,RN, "Terminal Agitation", *Journal of Hospice and Palliative Care Nursing* 2000; 2:1.
5. Johnston, Brian. "Deathly Quiet", World Net Daily, 4/13/02, available online at: http;//www.worldnetdaily.com/news/article/asp? ARTICLE_ID=227217
6. Kingsbury, Robert J., MD, "Palliative Sedation: May We Sleep Before We Die?" *Dignity* newsletter, Summer 2001.

Note. Other articles of interest can be found on the website of the Hospice Patients Alliance. http://www.hospicepatients.og/n-valko-terminal-sedation.html

Chapter 9

Abstinence From Food And Drink as a Means of Accelerating Death: The "Right to Die" Debate

Comments on a paper by Docker (1995) updated and reviewed by Craig

Introduction

In this review I will consider some issues as seen from the perspective of euthanasia activists, who advocate voluntary abstinence from food and drink as a means of accelerating death. My information is based on a paper written by Docker as published in 1995.[1] The paper as published in the journal 'The Dying in Dignity MENSA SIG NEW' in 1995, was brought to my attention in August 2003. It provides a useful review of early work in the field of hydration and nutrition at the end of life, but is heavily weighted with comments made from the perspective of advocates of euthanasia. Docker's article first appeared in 'Last Rights: Beyond Final Exit'.

The setting

The whole issue of withholding and withdrawing life prolonging medical treatment, including hydration and nutrition has become a battle ground for "Right to Die" activists, who do their best to influence legal judgements in their favour at legal test cases throughout the world. For example in the UK in 1996, the Voluntary Euthanasia Society backed Annie Lindsell, a motor neurone disease sufferer, in her unsuccessful court action.[2] More recently, in Australia in June 2003, a judgement in the Victoria Supreme Court permitted the withdrawal of tube feeding of a woman with severe pre-senile dementia, who was known only as BWV.[3] Pro-life groups were concerned about the judgement which they thought set a dangerous precedent.[4,5] Right to die activists on the other hand saw it as an act of political cowardice, for they argued that the patient should have been killed by delivery of a lethal dose of sedative through her feeding tube.[6] Since such an action is unlawful in most countries of the world, right to die activists have been campaigning for wider use of advance directives, to enable those seeking an exit from life to refuse life-prolonging treatment. As an alternative to advance directives or physician-assisted suicide, they advocate voluntary abstinence from food and drink- to bring about death by dehydration or starvation. The advantages and disadvantages of this course of action were considered by Docker in 1995.[1] His paper reviewed the situation from a predominantly North American viewpoint on the basis of articles published between 1950 and 1995.

Docker quoted from my paper in the Journal of Medical Ethics of 1994* and noted that I had failed to mention 'the rational self-deliverance of someone who has decided to end their own interminable and unrelievable suffering.' He redressed the balance by considering this issue at considerable length.

*See this book Chapter 2 page 9

Docker introduced his paper with the following statement:

"The right to die" debate as it affects patients and physicians, has taken a new and interesting turn in recent years in terms of rights, duties and co-operation. Abstinence from food and drink, as a means to willed, voluntary death, has been put forward as a solution to a particular legal and moral stalemate that has persisted between patients and doctors, right-to-die proponents and "pro-lifers".[1] For we see that

"...educating chronically ill and terminally ill patients about the feasibility of patient refusal of hydration and nutrition (PRHN) can empower them to control their own destiny without requesting physicians to reject their taboos on physician-assisted suicide (PAS) and voluntary assisted euthanasia (VAE) that have existed for millennia."[7] (Bernat, Gert and Mogielnicki 1993)

The evidence presented

Unfortunately for advocates of euthanasia, Docker noted that "This proposal, which seems to many an attractive one, is, however beleagured with apparently conflicting evidence about the painlessness of such a course of action...." Nevertheless on the basis of a review of literature available in 1995, he voiced the tentative and cautious conclusion that- "abstinence from food and drink as a means of accelerating death may be a viable method for suitable individuals, but our evidence suggests that, without medical examination of the person undergoing the fast to ascertain suitability, and the provision of palliative care to alleviate troubling symptoms, it may be an uncertain course for an individual to embark on..." [1]

Troublesome symptoms: the discomfort factor

Those reading the catalogue of symptoms and unpleasant effects of dehydration, fasting and starvation listed by Docker, would have to be very strong-minded indeed to starve or dehydrate themselves to death! On the basis of a survey of the published evidence from 1950 to 1994, Docker was inclined to take the view that many of the worrying comments made were 'emotionally laden', 'biased', 'irrational' or 'macabre'. Docker clearly dislikes medical science and dogmatic paternalism- for example he noted that " ... dogmatic paternalism occurs with increasing frequency when the problem is seen only in the (increasingly complex) language of medical science, and with an ear to medical science for the answer..." Perhaps he fears that science might undermine his attempt to present starvation and dehydration in a favourable light! Science may indeed prove that death from starvation or dehydration can be extremely unpleasant and uncomfortable. On the other hand, as I have discussed elsewhere, there is some evidence that thirst is indeed reduced in the frail elderly.[8] This point did not escape Docker, who mentioned the work of Phillips and Rolls.[9] While the jury is still out as regards thirst in dehydrated and dying cancer patients, there is little or no evidence to suggest that thirst reduction is a general feature of all dying patients.

Docker chose to ignore the work of Bruera and his colleagues in Canada who were exploring the value of hydration in terminally ill cancer patients in the early 1990s. They have since shown that maintenance of hydration reduces the incidence of terminal agitation markedly [10] - a point that must surely carry weight and swing opinion in favour of a more active approach to hydration in the years to come.

115

Evidence of benefit from dehydration

Docker struggled to find convincing evidence of the benefit, unless of course, death is considered to be a benefit. Nevertheless he drew attention to 1) anecdotal reports, 2) voluntary fasting as practised by a particular religious sect, the Jaina Digambura community, and 3) voluntary fasting in a hospital or hospice setting, including the withdrawal of nutrition and hydration at the request of competent patients. With regard to the third situation, Docker quoted an article by Ahronheim and Gasner in the Lancet of 1990 [11] as saying that 'Withholding or withdrawing artificial feeding and hydration from debilitated patients does not result in a gruesome, cruel or violent death...deprivation of fluid rapidly results in further depression of consciousness, and then coma... There is also some evidence that impaired thirst may occur naturally with advanced age or neurological impairment, and that there may be endogenous production of substances producing natural analgesia.' [11]

The issue of starvation

Docker discussed this at some length, and listed many references. He referred to the early work of Keys describing his paper as 'a classic'. [12] Keys reported some apparent geographical differences in the effects of starvation, for example certain problems were not uncommon in the Orient, but exceedingly rare in modern Europe. Others, such as nutritional neuropathies were more prevalent in tropical and semi-tropical regions. Thus the situation is extremely complex.

Naturally when advocating voluntary abstinence from food and drink as a means of accelerating death, euthanasia activists play down the problems and discomfort. However when it comes to withholding and withdrawing fluids and sustenance from patients such as BWV, the Australian lady with pre-senile dementia they emphasise the drawbacks and discomfort. Commenting on the ruling in the case of BWV in May 2003, Dr Rodney Syme, president of the Voluntary Euthanasia Society of Victoria, noted that the "...Supreme Court ruling that a guardian with the ability to refuse sustenance could be appointed for a woman in a vegetative state is a milestone, but one that commits her to a macabre death...her family can now decide to remove the tube... This will lead to death by dehydration and starvation, possibly taking two to three weeks. Would you inflict this form of slow death on your pet? No? Then why must a human suffer like this?" Syme argued that a lethal dose of sedative down the tube would be preferable, and described euthanasia as "a palliative act and, for many people, the optimal choice of palliation." [6] Sadly this view of palliation was given credence by Billings, an American Palliative Care Physician at Massachusetts General Hospital, for writing in the British Medical Journal in 2000 he discussed physician-assisted suicide as if it was simply an aspect of palliative care! [13]

Legal issues

At an early stage in his paper, Docker noted that patients have the right to refuse life-support systems, such as 'forced feeding by gastric tubes, and intravenous drips of expensive nutrient solutions. They also have the right to palliative care.' [14] However please note, that in some enlightened corners of the world, for example in the State of Victoria, Australia, palliative care used to include 'the reasonable provision of food and water which is not burdensome to the patient'. [5] Nevertheless in the recent case of BWV, a woman with pre-senile dementia, the judge defined tube feeding as medical treatment, and allowed it to be withdrawn, to the great concern of many commentators.[3,4] The Archbishop of Melbourne commented "…It is clear that this is what the euthanasia lobby wanted. They know- as every health professional knows- that law and medicine already allow the withdrawal of inappropriate forms of care. But euthanasia advocates have been looking for a test case with which to get the courts drastically to alter the laws protecting human life…" [5] The case of BWV is, to the State of Victoria, what the Bland case was to England and Wales.

With respect to the Bland case of 1993 that left our law 'misshapen', Docker mentions an interesting comment made at that time by Lord Mustill, namely that "…in 20 out of 39 American states which have legalised in favour of 'Living wills' the legislation specifically excludes terminating life by the withdrawal of nourishment and hydration." [15] Thus the measures that Docker and right-to-die activists are trying to promote are of dubious legality. This however does not bother the Voluntary Euthanasia Society, for their aim is to change the law.

Some views from the literature

During the course of his paper Docker quoted a number of interesting but conflicting views from the literature, for example-

- *75% of physicians surveyed objected to the idea of withdrawing fluids. (Thomasma, Micetich and Steinecker 1986)* [16]
- *Physicians frequently regard fluids and food to be minimum standards of care for the dying. (ibid 1986)* [16]
- *'The only medically secure treatment for a dying patient is comfort. That is the only way medicine can benefit such persons. We have argued that nutrition and fluids are optional treatments on this basis.' (ibid 1986)* [16]
- *'A social decision to permit physicians or health care facilities to deny food and fluids to patients who are capable of receiving and utilizing them, directly attacks the very foundation of medicine as an ethical profession.' (Derr 1986)* [17]
- *'No matter how simple, inexpensive, readily available, non-invasive, and common the procedure, if it does not offer substantial hope of benefit to the patient, he has no moral obligation to undergo it, nor the physician to provide it, nor the judge to order it.' (Paris J.1986)* [18]
- *'For physicians, provision of ordinary means of comfort and care- like food and water- demonstrates our personal, professional, and social commitment to the dying patient.' (Siegler 1987)* [19]
- *Docker accepted the simplistic and contested view propounded by many palliative carers, namely that 'Discomfort from dehydration may be entirely absent as long as the mouth is kept moist.' (Billings 1985)* [20]
- *'…the assumption in the argument, that the dying must be hungry and thirsty, has not been proved. Indeed, as has been noted, the opposite is suspected by many who have worked closely with the dying.' (Printz 1992)* [21]
- *'In the literature, the issue of medical hydration and nutrition in the dying patient remains one of the underexplored areas of medicine' (Printz 1992)* [21]

Conclusions

Docker concluded that 'As death from lack of nutrition alone is a potentially very lengthy process, a combination of ceasing nutrition and hydration by some method is likely to be a preferred course. This area undoubtedly needs much more research. While a peaceful death by this method seems feasible in some instances, without particularized medical advice and medical backup, and until more is known about the process of self-deliverance this way, an isolated individual, on available data, would appear to have greater assurance of success by means of drugs.

Thus somewhat tentatively, Docker and right-to-die activists advocate suicide by self-induced dehydration and starvation or a lethal overdose of drugs. It would in my view be entirely unethical for a doctor to encourage a patient to take this course of action, or to assist them in any way. Physician-assisted suicide remains unlawful in the United Kingdom and in most states of the USA. It is a basic principle of medical ethics that "The doctor may use his professional knowledge only to improve or maintain the health of those who put their trust in him; in no circumstances may he act to their detriment." [22]

Acknowledgement and note. Mr Docker is currently the Director of Exit, an organisation that was formerly known as the Voluntary Euthanasia Society of Scotland. In 1995 Docker was their Executive Secretary. He has an M. Phil. in Law and Ethics in Medicine, and is particularly interested in 'self-deliverance' (suicide). Dr Craig thanks Mr Chris Docker for permission to quote from his paper, but does not share his views.

References

1   Docker C. Abstinence from food and drink as a means of accelerating death. *Dignity in Dying. Mensa Special Interest Group News* 1995; **12 (1)** :31-41. © C. Docker. Quoted with permission.

2   Dyer C. Court confirms right to palliative treatment for mental distress. *British Medical Journal*;1997; **315**:1178.

3   Fisher A. We're all dying for an answer. *Herald Sun.* (Melbourne) June 2nd. 2003.

4   Perrin D. End-of-life decisions: the moral issues at stake. *AD2000*, August 2003, p6.

5   Westmore P. Archbishop Hart defends woman in euthanasia case. *AD2000*, July 2003, p3. © AD2000. Quoted with permission.

6   Syme R. Put heat on our MPs. *Herald Sun.* May 30th 2003.

7   Bernat J., Gert B., Mogielnicki R. Patient refusal of hydration and nutrition. *Archives of Internal Medicine*, 1993; **153**: 2723-2728, p2723. Quoted with permission.

8   Craig GM. Death from dehydration: some pros and cons. *Catholic Medical Quarterly* May 2001.

9   Phillips P, Rolls BJ, Ledingham JGG et al. Reduced thirst after water deprivation in healthy elderly men. *New England Journal of Medicine* 1984; **311**: 753-9.

10 Bruera E, Franco JJ, Maltoni M et al. Changing pattern of agitated impaired mental status in patients with advanced cancer: association with cognitive monitoring, hydration, and opioid rotation. *Journal of Pain and Symptom Management*, 1995; **10**: 287-291.

11 Ahronheim J, Gasner M. The sloganism of starvation. *Lancet* 1990; **335**:278-279.

12 Keys A, Brozek J, Henschel A, Mickelson O, Taylor H. The Biology of Human Starvation 1&11. Minneapolis; *University of Minnesota Press* 1950, 1:583-4.

13 Billings JA, Recent advances in palliative care. *British Medical Journal*, 2000; **321**: 555-558.

14 Frederick G. An easy alternative to assisted suicide. *Globe and Mail*, 1993, September 3rd. p A 19.

15 Lord Mustill. Airedale NHS Trust v Bland [1993] 1.All ER, 820, 888.

16 Thomasma D, Micetich K, Steinecker P, "Continuance of Nutritional Care in the Terminally Ill Patient" *Critical Care Clinics* 1986; **2(1)**: 61-71. Quoted with permission from Elsevier.

17 Derr P. Why food and fluids can never be denied. *Hastings Centre Report* 1986; **16(1)**: 28-30. © Quoted with permission.

18 Paris J. When burdens of feeding outweigh benefits. *Hastings Centre Report* 1986; **16(1)**; 30-32. © Quoted with permission.

19 Siegler M, Schiedermeyer D, Should fluid and nutritional support be withheld from terminally ill patients?- Tube feeding in hospice settings. *American Journal of Hospice Care*. 1987 March/April 32-35, at 35.

20 Billings J. Comfort measures for the terminally ill: is dehydration painful? *Journal of the American Geriatrics Society* 1985; **33(11):** 808-810.

21 Printz L. Terminal dehydration, a compassionate treatment. *Archives of Internal Medicine* 1992; **152**: 697-700. © Quoted with permission.

22 Principles of Medical Ethics in Europe. 1987, Article 2. Quoted by Irish Medical Council 1995. See ref 21. Craig. Journal of Medical Ethics 1996, **22**: 147-153.

Chapter 10

An International Perspective

1. American palliative care as portrayed by Billings

Reviewed by Gillian Craig.

Those who wish to read about current concepts in palliative care as seen from the perspective of an American palliative care specialist, may find an article by J. Andrew Billings illuminating.[1] It was published in the British Medical Journal in September 2000 and coincided, by chance or design, with a conference of the World Federation of Right-to -Die Societies, held in Boston, Massachusetts in September 2000. Sadly it seems that events in the USA have been influenced not one iota by the hydration debate as launched in the Journal of Medical Ethics in 1994. It receives no mention, yet Billings claims to have reviewed advances in palliative care over the last five years. The favoured approach in the USA appears to be to let the patient die and to bring this about by withholding hydration, through the patient's contemporaneous choice, or by advance directives or proxy decision makers if the patient is mentally incompetent.

Billings argues that dehydration in advanced illness 'does not seem to cause physical discomfort, and need not be treated or prevented with artificial hydration.' He bases this view on the work of McCann and colleagues as published in 1994,[2] yet this work is deeply flawed and does not stand up to critical scrutiny.

The paper by McCann and colleagues was a study of 32 elderly patients in a terminal care unit in the USA. They were given food and fluids on request, and were capable, at least initially, of expressing sensations of hunger and thirst. No artificial alimentation or hydration was used. Most patients had terminal cancer. One had sustained a stroke. Approximately two thirds of the patients (66%) experienced thirst for the first 25% of their stay. One third (33%) felt thirsty until they died, and one third (33%) experienced no thirst and continued to be able to drink. The symptom of thirst was relieved for variable lengths of time, ranging from one hour to several hours, by mouth toilet and, in some cases, drinks. Crucially no attempt was made to sort out whether thirst relief was shorter in those on mouth toilet only, than in those who could drink. Physiologically one would expect prolonged thirst relief only in those who swallowed significant amounts of fluids, as expounded by Verbalis whose work I have mentioned already.[3]

McCann and colleagues state that 'It is probable that most of our patients died with dehydration ....' which as they point out can cloud the senses to the point of coma. Only one patient in the study had a food and fluid intake deemed to be more than 75% sufficient. The authors were aware of defects in their study, namely:

1   Lack of controls.
2   Staff assessments of comfort may have been biased.
3   Levels of comfort and suffering were difficult to assess.
4   Narcotic use may have masked symptoms.

Much was made of the potential adverse effects of artificial nutrition aggressively applied. No mention was made of the possibility of relieving dehydration by subcutaneous fluids. McCann's flawed paper confirms that thirst is a significant symptom in many terminally ill patients, and that dehydration is often left untreated. To use the data to justify withholding artificial hydration is completely unwarranted.

The 'hospice approach' to dementia care in a specialist dementia unit in the USA resulted in 62% of patients dying with the lowest level of supportive care, a result that Billings found 'remarkable'. Equally remarkable to my way of thinking was the fact that Billings discussed physician assisted suicide for terminally ill people as if it was simply an aspect of palliative care. It is no such thing! Physician assisted suicide remains illegal in all American States except Oregon. As Billings acknowledged it is time to shift discussion to other issues.

Sadly some commentators in the USA encourage people to stop eating and drinking as an alternative to physician assisted suicide, and others endorse the practice of sedation without hydration for the relief of otherwise intractable suffering in a dying patient - references are given by Billings.

I note that Derek Doyle, an influential and senior British palliative care specialist, made many suggestions on the paper in its final revision, yet no mention was made of our national guidelines on the ethical use of artificial hydration in terminally ill patients. This regrettable omission leads me to suspect that poor publicity given to these guidelines was intentional. The publication of Billings' paper in the British Medical Journal can be seen as another attempt to bury the hydration debate!

Futile Care Theory based on the concept of 'comfort care only' is far advanced in the United States of America. Wesley J. Smith, a perceptive attorney based in California, has warned that 'All over the country, in hospitals, nursing homes and other facilities, conscious but cognitively disabled and aged people are being denied adequate care and/or being starved and dehydrated to death in the name of patient autonomy, "quality of life" and "best interest of the patient" determinations…'[4] This comment demonstrates what is happening in the USA to people who are not imminently dying, whose lives could be prolonged for a significant length of time by measures such as tube feeding or antibiotics for treatable infections. The American approach to 'managed death' will prevail in the UK soon, unless wiser counsel prevails.

References

1   Billings JA. Recent advances in palliative care. *British Medical Journal.* 2000; **321**: 555-558.

2   McCann RM. Hall WJ. Groth-Juncker A. Comfort care for terminally ill patients: the appropriate use of nutrition and hydration. *Journal of the American Medical Association.* 1994; **272**: 1263-6.

3   Verbalis JG. 1991. His figure © Springer-Verlag was reprinted with permission in an article by Craig , *Ethics & Medicine.* 1999; **15:1**; p17 and is reproduced on page 103 of this book.

4   Smith. W.J. Creating a disposable caste. San Francisco Chronicle. December 8th 1995.

2. Science, hospice, and terminal dehydration

Author Steven Baumrucker, M.D.

This article was first published in the American Journal of Hospice & Palliative Care, Volume 16, Number 3, pp 502-3 in May/June 1999. The author is Associate Editor-in-Chief of that journal. Reprinted with permission.
© Prime National Publishing Corporation, 470 Boston Post Road, Weston, MA 02493.

Hospice care as a science is a relatively new discipline. Literary references to hospice-type care can be found as far back as Shakespeare (see *Henry V* and the care Falstaff received at end-of-life from his cohort at the inn), but "palliative care" was not referred to as such. Symptom control was merely the standard-of-care in times before modern medicine brought an expectation of cure or modification of the natural history of the disease. What else could the early practitioner offer in most cases, but palliation of symptoms?

To bring science to the care of patients at end-of-life has been a long process, and one that is still in its infancy. This lack of evidence-based data encourages the "art" of palliative medicine, but makes decision-making more difficult, especially to the new or part-time practitioner. An artful practitioner is a joy to behold, and his or her patients are lucky indeed, but transmitting "art" to the next generation of practitioners is harder and less efficient than transmitting evidence-based decision-making.

For example, there are a few studies examining the use of nebulized morphine for terminal dyspnoea. The most positive studies are unblended, observational studies, [1] while the most negative study is a blinded, placebo-controlled series in a *non-hospice population*.[2] Physiologic studies were done on cows.[3] From this scattered evidence, the practitioner must somehow make a clinical decision when and if to use nebulized opioids in the setting of terminal dyspnoea.

The question of dehydration in the terminally ill is a similar, although possibly better studied, minefield. Even the most accomplished researchers in the field conclude " the data reported to date are insufficient to allow a final conclusion on the benefit or harm of dehydration in terminally ill patients." [4] Research has indicated that fluid depletion in dying patients is at least relatively benign in symptoms, and that comfort levels can be maintained, even when dehydration is such that the serum sodium levels become deranged.[5] However Fainsinger showed that delirium could be significantly decreased at end-of-life if severe dehydration was avoided with a small amount (approximately 1200cc/day) of administered fluids.[4]

Whenever we wish to try a new intervention, we involve the patient or family in the decision-making process. When we, as deliverers of health care, are not certain what the best course of treatment is we often defer the decision to the patient or family, assessing their comfort level with one direction versus another (this can also be referred to as "dumping it in their laps"). Patient attitudes, level of comfort with the situation, and education will influence the decision; health care workers attitudes, level of education, and biases in presentation ("You don't want me to give IV fluids, do you?") will also affect the outcome. To know what factors are relevant to patients' acceptance or denial of hydration will show us how to better approach the situation when it arises; if a certain identifiable population of patients nearly always refuse terminal hydration, then one could spend more time on other interventions and less energy pushing an unacceptable modality.

The article by Morita *et al.* in this issue [6] takes a step towards defining what factors enter the decision for or against hydration at the end-of-life by patients and family. The study is well discussed in the body of the article, but a few points are very interesting, although not truly part of the study.

First, most impressive is that over 90 percent of family members participated in the decision whether to hydrate. Fifty one percent of patients also participated; the rest were felt to be too delirious. In contrast, one Israeli study showed that only three percent of patients and 13 percent of families participated in a similar decision on an oncology ward.[7] The average in the Unites States is probably somewhere in the middle. The level of participation in Japan, if the results can be generalized, is stunning and should be emulated elsewhere.

Also amazing is the statement "...more than half of the care-receivers stated that...artificial fluid therapy might worsen patient's suffering." In this country, where we usually only feel comfortable when we are "doing something," it is unlikely that one could find 51 percent of health care practitioners who would agree with this enlightened view, much less 51 percent of the population at large. How the Japanese public seemingly became so familiar with an issue that is foreign to ours is an interesting question. Is it all cultural, and therefore not transferable here, or is there a way that we can educate ourselves and our clients so that they can make more rational decisions about their own fates when we necessarily defer to them for guidance?

To be able to say something like "studies have shown, that in this instance, the majority of patients feel better if we don't give them fluids" works reasonably well in this society. Perhaps this is just another reason to encourage the scientific pursuit of answers to questions at the end-of-life. If we can use science to further the art of delivering health care, part of which is helping patients and families make decisions with a minimum of stress, then we have at least achieved symmetry. At best, we will decrease suffering, which is the reason our specialty exists.

References

1   Farncombe: *Palliative Medicine*. 1994; **8**: 306.
2   Noseda A: *Euro Resp J.* 1997; **10**: 1079.
3   Zappi L: Opioid agonists modulate release of neurotransmitters in bovine trachealis muscle. *Anesthesiology*. 1995; **83 (3):** 543.
4   Fainsinger RL, Bruera E: When to treat dehydration in a terminally ill patient? *Support Care Cancer*. 1997; **5 (3):**205.
5   Nullo-navich K, et al.: Comfort and incidence of abnormal serum sodium, BUN, creatinine and osmolality in dehydration of terminal illness. *American Journal of Hospice and Palliative Care*. 1998; **15(2):** 77-84.
6   Morita T, et al.: Perceptions and decision- making on rehydration of terminally ill cancer patients and family members. *American Journal of Hospice and Palliative Care*. 1999; **16(3):** 509-516.

7   Musgrave CF, et al.: Intravenous hydration for terminal patients: What are the attitudes of Israeli terminal patients, their families, and their health care professionals? *Journal of Pain and Symptom Management.* 1996; **12**: 47.

3. Factors that influence decisions about rehydration of terminally ill cancer patients.

A study from Japan by Morita, Tsuonoda, Inoue and Chihara in 1999
Reviewed by Gillian Craig

Morita, Tsunoda, Inoue and Chihara have studied how the perceptions of Japanese hospice patients and their families influence their decisions about the use of artificial hydration in terminally ill cancer patients. Their interesting paper was published in the American Journal of Hospice and Palliative Care in 1999 [1].

When explaining the reasons for their work Morita et al. referred to the debate in the Journal of Medical Ethics and to a range of papers on hydration and/or nutrition in terminal cancer patients. They noted that there was conflicting evidence about the indications for rehydration therapy in palliative care settings, and took the view that clinical decisions should depend on the preference of the patient and their family. This accords with the culture of Japan where the family plays a great role in decision-making. The aim of the study was to identify the factors that contributed to decisions to give or withhold artificial hydration once patients could no longer maintain a satisfactory oral intake.

Morita et al. undertook a prospective study of 121 consecutive terminally ill cancer patients who were admitted to the Seirei Hospice attached to a hospital in Japan. When patients could no longer drink enough, a physician explained the medical situation to them and to their family. In general the physicians advised against rehydration if there was evidence of severe fluid retention or physical suffering, but were not averse to rehydration in patients with a fair condition and tolerable symptoms. Having explained the situation, and made recommendations, the physicians carried out a structured interview. This posed several leading questions such as 'Do you believe that rehydration prolongs meaningless life? .... Do you believe withholding rehydration leads to premature death? .... Do you believe rehydration deteriorated patients' symptoms? .... Do you believe that withholding rehydration deteriorates patients' symptoms?' .... And so on. Various other factors that may have contributed to decision-making were also recorded. The patient's general condition was measured on a scale of 0 to 100 using the Palliative Care Performance Scale that runs from normal (100) to death (0).[2] The majority of patients (62%) were at the bottom end of the scale at 10-20, and nearing death. Almost half the patients (59 in all) were unable to contribute to discussion because of delirium (n=48) or dementia (n=11). Two had no competent family members. Thus the survey was based on interviews with 62 patients and 119 family members.

Various complicated multiple logistic regression analyses were undertaken on the data using a computer programme. Analysis showed in general that the views of the patients and their families corresponded closely with the physician's advice about rehydration, but in a small percentage of cases patients and/or their families went against medical advice. Overall 25% of patients received artificial hydration and 75% did not. In the majority of cases medical advice was accepted despite reservations and anxiety about the outcome. It was noted that some patients seemed hesitant to answer honestly. The results could be taken to indicate that patients and their relatives remained ambivalent and seriously concerned about the outcome regardless of whether hydration was given or not. Their main concerns were related to nutrition, survival and the patient's distress.

The main factors that deterred physicians from recommending rehydration were a poor condition on the Palliative Performance Scale (PPS) and the presence of severe fluid retention, as indicated by symptomatic pleural effusion, ascites or peripheral oedema. These medical terms indicate collections of fluid that are outside the circulatory system, in the chest, the abdomen or peripheral tissues. The causes are multifactorial and do not necessarily indicate fluid overload within the circulatory system. The authors do not say whether the patients had a raised venous pressure or unequivocal evidence of cardiac failure, which might of course be a very good reason for limiting the fluid intake. On the other hand, a pleural effusion or ascites may be an inflammatory response to cancer cells, in which case fluid restriction would not necessarily be appropriate. Every patient must be assessed individually. Good clinical judgement is essential for good medical care.

In discussion the authors mention other studies in the literature and come to the conclusion that the usual reasons given for rehydration are the need to give food and water, preservation of life, symptom palliation, "not giving up" and anxiety release. On the other hand they note that the main reasons for withholding hydration are said to be concern about dependency, becoming a burden, or prolonging suffering. In support of these statements they refer to the work of Holden [3] on the emotional impact of anorexia on terminally ill cancer patients and the family, and note a study by Meares [4]. They also draw on the work of Musgrave from Israel, where very few family members are included in decision-making [5] and note a paper by Parkash and Burge.[6] These references can be followed up by those who wish to explore this topic in greater depth.

The Japanese workers admit that their findings have not resolved the questions they have raised. Their work underlines how difficult it is to study complex and emotive issues in the dying. They make the important observation that there have been no controlled trials on the effects of simple rehydration therapy on the prognosis of terminally ill cancer patients. They also note that with the exception of thirst and delirium, the effect of rehydration on most symptoms has not been investigated. Nevertheless, on the basis of limited evidence, they take the conventional view that '....rehydration for terminal patients with extremely poor general condition is not appropriate unless they suffer from agitated delirium.'

Baumrucker, commenting on the work of Morita wondered how the Japanese public were able to say that artificial fluid therapy might worsen patient's suffering – a view that he described as 'enlightened'.[7] I venture to suggest that the family members did not know but deferred to the opinion of the hospice medical staff. Without evidence it is premature to describe this view as "enlightened". The truth is that no one really knows until further research is done.

Morita et al. rightly concluded that further studies on the effect of rehydration on patient's survival and distress should be strongly encouraged. They also recognised the need for further studies that focus attention on family concerns about rehydration and the relationship between these concerns and psychological distress.

References

1 Morita T, Tsunoda J, Inoue S and Chihara S. Perceptions and decision-making on rehydration of terminally ill cancer patients and family members. *American Journal of Hospice and Palliative Care.* 1999; **16:** 509-516.

2 Anderson F, Downing GM, Hill J. Palliative Performance Scale. (PPS): A new tool. *Journal of Palliative Care.* 1996; **12:** 5-11.

3 Holden CM. Anorexia in terminally ill cancer patients. The emotional impact on the patient and family. *Hospital Journal.* 1991; **7:** 73-84.

4 Meares CJ. Primary care giver perceptions of intake cessation in patients who are terminally ill. Oncology Nurses Forum. 1997; **24:** 1751-56.

5 Musgrave CF, Bartral N, Opstad J. Intravenous hydration for terminal patients. What are the attitudes of Israeli terminal patients, their families and their health care professionals? *Journal of Pain and Symptom Management.* 1996; **12:** 47-51.

6 Parkash R, Burge F. The family's perspective on issues of hydration in terminal care. *Journal of Palliative Care.* 1997; **13:** 23-27.

7 Baumrucker S. Science, hospice, and terminal dehydration. *American Journal of Hospice and Palliative Care.*1999; **16:** 502-3.

4. Palliative care in Australia

Views expressed by Ashby and Stoffell have been presented and discussed at some length already in the course of the debate.[1] Clearly there are centres of excellence in Australia where traditional palliative care of the highest quality is practiced. Elsewhere there is cause for concern as indicated by the following case that came to court.

The case of John Thompson of Sidney [2]

John Thompson was 37 years old and single on March 2nd 2000 when he had a cardiac arrest following a heroin overdose and was admitted unconscious to the Royal Prince Alfred Hospital (RPAH). Within a matter of days he had been written off, as a person for whom there was no hope and was transferred from the intensive care unit to a renal transplant ward. He developed a lung infection and was thought to have irreversible brain damage. A "Not for Resuscitation Order" (NFR) was issued against the wishes of the relatives. When his 80 year old mother asked the Consultant not to take him off antibiotics her request was refused on grounds of futility, and an adverse neurological report. When he developed a raging fever his sister's request for assistance from the nursing staff was met with a display of annoyance. The story has a familiar ring to it! However Australians appear to be able to access help from the law with admirable speed! Thanks to a phone call from the patient's sister Mrs Northridge

(Mrs N.) the Duty Judge in the New South Wales Supreme Court heard of the case on Sunday March 12th. By that time the patient was on morphine, antibiotics and intravenous fluids had been stopped, and death was inevitable without urgent intervention. Mrs N. sought an order to prevent the RPAH from withdrawing treatment and life support from her brother. With admirable speed the Duty Judge formulated 14 questions, contacted the Duty Security Officer, dictated them to him and asked him to submit them to Mrs N. and get her replies as soon as possible. By 3.25pm that day the Duty Security Officer telephoned the Judge with the answers. The Judge then contacted the Hospital Registrar who was at her home. She confirmed that if treatment was not maintained and if the patient was not fed, he would die. The Judge then informed the doctor that unless some accommodation could be reached it would be necessary to have a hearing later that evening. He asked her to "consider the maintenance of the status quo, by giving antibiotics to the patient and feeding intravenously." The Registrar advised the Consultant of the position and he agreed to resume treatment. The matter was then listed for attention in Court the following morning. The Judge Mr Justice O'Keefe took the trouble to contact the appropriate officer of the Central Sydney Area Health Service to advise him of the proposed hearing, and asked him to contact the RPAH's solicitor or the Crown Solicitor.

Those of us who know how exceedingly difficult it can be to obtain legal support in the UK will be amazed by the speed and efficiency of the New South Wales Supreme Court.

The Judge was exercising an ancient *parens patriae jurisdiction*- this being "The jurisdiction to protect the person of those who are not able to do so themselves..." In so doing the Judge made it clear that "the paramount consideration is to preserve the life of or safeguard, secure or promote, or prevent the deterioration in the physical or mental health of the subject..." in accordance with the principle of necessity. Consequently any "treatment or other procedures undertaken must be in the best interests of preserving the life, health or welfare of the person concerned." Australian Courts recognise that the exercise of this jurisdiction "should not be for the benefit of others...including a health care system that is intent on saving on costs..." [2]

Following the intervention of the court antibiotic treatment and feeding were reinstated, the NFR order was revoked, and a gradual reduction in morphine dose was introduced. On the 20th of March the patient had a respiratory arrest, was ventilated and recovered. Had the NFR order still been in place he would have died. On April 12th there was some discussion between the family and a neurologist regarding what action to take in the event of another cardiac arrest. The neurologist was in favour of doing nothing, but Mrs N. did not agree. She arranged for a further opinion from two distinguished independent neurologists. When examined by Professor James Lance on April 30th. the patient was alert and moved his limbs on request, but could not speak as he had a tracheotomy. His condition had clearly improved markedly since admission. The Professor expected him to improve further to a point where he could swallow and speak. The second neurologist Dr Edward Freeman a Consultant for the National Brain Injury Foundation, saw the patient on April 28th. He was of the opinion that a premature diagnosis of 'chronic vegetative state' had been made, and recommended active rehabilitation for six months. Moreover he concluded that what had occurred in relation to Mr John Thompson was not a rare case. In his experience "...the discarding of people with severe brain injury by the health care system in Australia, unfortunately is very familiar... and very frustrating."[2]

Thanks to the intervention of the court, the patient survived, and was in due course moved to a nursing home. He can move, respond, write, and articulate. By a strange irony the patient was saved by a Judge who was prepared to invoke the doctrine of necessity, a doctrine that we are in danger of abandoning in the UK.

References

1. Ashby M, and Stoffell B. Journal of medical ethics 1995; **21**: 135-140.
2. Northridge v Central Sydney Area Health Service [2000] NSWSC 1241 (29 December 2000)

Chapter 11
Rehydration in Terminally Ill Patients

1. The technical possibilities

When a person is unable to take fluids by mouth, hydration can be maintained by the use of an intravenous drip, by fluids given by the subcutaneous route, or via a nasogastric tube, or, on occasions, by the rectal route. Fluids *and* nutrition can be given via a nasogastric tube or via a tube that enters the stomach through the abdominal wall, or on rare occasions by the risky technique of total parenteral nutrition. In general the more invasive the technique, the greater the reluctance to use it in a person who is terminally ill. If the means of administration of hydration or nutrition is considered too great a burden for the patient to bear, it is ethical and right to refrain from intervention.

Professor Eduardo Bruera and his colleagues in Canada have been leading advocates of hydration in terminally ill cancer patients for a number of years. In late 1990, it became standard practice on the palliative care unit at Edmonton General Hospital in Alberta, to monitor patients for delirium and to treat affected patients with artificial hydration and opioid rotation (i.e. changing the type of morphine given). These simple interventions reduced the incidence of agitated delirium markedly – in fact by two thirds. This is a very important observation since, as Bruera points out, agitated delirium is a devastating experience for the patient, the family, and health-care staff. It is also, in Bruera's experience, the most common cause of conflict between the staff and the patient's family.[1]

The subcutaneous route for fluid administration has many potential advantages over the intravenous route in patients who do not need large volumes of fluids or close monitoring of electrolytes. In most cases fluids can be given with less discomfort and cost than by the intravenous route. The technique can be used in nursing homes or in the patient's own home, since close supervision by health care staff is not required.[2]

In isolated rural areas or developing countries where access to medical and nursing care is limited and sterile needles, tubes and fluids hard to come by or too expensive, there is a place for the use of tap water given via a fine tube into the rectum. Bruera finds this method safe, effective, cheap and quite well tolerated by patients [3]. Most however, would prefer subcutaneous hydration where that option exists. Nevertheless, a slow overnight drip of tap water into the rectum – "this homely remedy" – as described by Wilkes may still have a place, and could well be preferable to death from dehydration.

Hydration alone cannot sustain life. In the absence of food, if dehydration is prevented, death from starvation will occur within 60 days.

2. The need for nutrition

The average length of time that a patient dying of cancer needs artificial hydration is 14 days, so the question of maintaining nutrition will rarely arise in a hospice setting.

However, if swallowing difficulties develop when death is not imminent, the need for nutrition as well as hydration, must be addressed. The situation will vary according to the pathology and the long term outlook. The medical team may need to consider measures such as feeding via a nasogastric tube, or a tube placed in the stomach via the abdominal wall. The latter is called percutaneous endoscopic gastrostomy (PEG for short). This might be appropriate for example, in some patients with swallowing difficulties due to malignancies in the mouth or throat, and in patients with neurological disorders such as strokes and motor neurone disease. In skilled hands a PEG can be introduced quite simply in 10-30 minutes under local anaesthetic plus intravenous sedation. The mortality of the procedure is less than 1%. The benefits and risks of a PEG should be considered carefully in patients who need tube feeding for longer than six weeks. A PEG has certain aesthetic advantages over a nasogastric tube since it is invisible under clothing. It is also more efficient than a nasogastric tube. For further information see an excellent article in Geriatric Medicine.[4]

Where the gut is not capable of absorbing food, for example in intestinal obstruction, it is possible to maintain nutrition by means of special nutrient solutions given into a major vein. This technique, known as total parenteral nutrition (TPN), is used when the pathology is potentially reversible or when nutritional deficit from a non-malignant cause is life threatening. An example of the first situation might be a patient with intestinal obstruction due to a tumour that may respond to chemotherapy (e.g. cancer of the ovary). An example of the second would be an individual who had lost a critical amount of intestinal absorptive capacity through disease, such as Crohn's disease. TPN requires a high level of skilled medical supervision and is never undertaken lightly.

Some people may question the need to discuss the use of a PEG or TPN in a book about hydration in terminal care. However, terminal illness has been defined as follows by the NHS Executive and the National Council for Hospice and Specialist Palliative Care Services in London:- "Terminally ill people are those with active and progressive disease for which curative treatment is not possible or not appropriate, and from which death can reasonably be expected within 12 months."[5] Given this time scale, the nutritional needs of terminally ill patients cannot be overlooked, even in a palliative care setting. An excellent state of the art paper on the assessment of nutritional status and fluid deficits in advanced cancer was published recently.[6]

It is becoming increasingly clear that to withhold hydration or nutrition with the deliberate intention of causing death is unlawful. This should go without saying, but these days it is necessary to restate this fact. Professor Gillon, writing in the British Medical Journal recently, said – "We all have a *prima facie* moral obligation not to intend our patients' deaths ... we must never treat our patients with the intention of accelerating their deaths."[7]

If food and water is regarded as a basic human need, rather than "treatment", doctors might pay more attention to hydration and nutrition in terminal care. To maintain hydration is a relatively simple matter as the papers from Bruera and colleagues show. To maintain nutrition in a person who cannot eat normally is quite a different story. The risks of maintaining nutrition by invasive means must be taken into a very careful consideration by the medical team. The feasibility of intervention via a PEG and the wisdom of embarking on TPN, requires a skilled medical judgement. Insertion of a PEG or TPN tube is a skilled medical procedure. However, once inserted, a PEG enables a patient to be nourished quite simply and without discomfort. Those who insert PEGs regularly, regard their use as a normal part of patient care. Those with less experience are more reluctant to consider them. As with all technological procedures involved in life support, they should be used with discretion.

In the final analysis, the issue for medical and nursing staff should be primarily one of practicalities. Does intervention "offer a reasonable chance of an appreciable duration of desirable life at an acceptable cost of suffering?"[8] The difficult elements in the question can only be answered by the medical team involved, in close liaison with the patient and/or their nearest and dearest friends or relatives.

Medical teams and relatives should be wary of making negative decisions about intervention, without consulting the patient. In a survey of 23 hospice patients with incurable and advanced malignancy, 11 requested cardiopulmonary resuscitation in the event of a cardiac arrest, whereas their key nurse would have considered this inappropriate. "Perhaps", wrote Meystre, Ahmedzai and Burley, "the most important lesson is that even a terminally ill patient with an incurable malignancy may find life worthwhile and precious." [9]

In matters of hydration and nutrition, palliative care staff should discuss the options with the patients and listen to their wishes.

Fainsinger and Bruera take issue with palliative care colleagues who are strongly opposed to using drips and argue that 'the viewpoint that dehydration in dying patients is not a cause of symptom distress overlooks commonly reported problems, such as agitated delirium, that can be prevented or reversed by the management of dehydration...' However having reviewed the evidence available in 1997 they commented that 'the data reported to date are insufficient to allow a final conclusion on the benefit or harm of dehydration in terminally ill patients. Nevertheless, it is worth considering that while some dying patients may not suffer any ill effects from dehydration, there may be others who do manifest symptoms, such as confusion or opioid toxicity, that might be alleviated or prevented by parenteral hydration.' [10]

3. Rehydration in palliative and terminal care: if not why not?

This crucial question was the subject of an important paper that was published in the journal Palliative Medicine in 1995.[11] The lead authors Kilean Dunphy and Ilora Finlay had chaired the ethics committee of the Association for Palliative Medicine of Great Britain and Northern Ireland at an early stage in the debate. Ilora Finlay set the ball rolling in 1994 on receipt of a reprint of my initial article in the Journal of Medical Ethics, and was succeeded later by Kilean Dunphy, who debated the issues with me at a conference at the Royal College of Physicians in 1997 and unveiled the National Council (NCSHPCS) guidelines on the ethical use of artificial hydration.[12]

The views expressed by Dunphy, Finlay *et al* can be taken to reflect discussion that preceded publication of the guidelines. The authors reviewed the evidence on rehydration in palliative and terminal care and challenged their colleagues 'to admit our uncertainty, to make genuine and unprejudged assessments of the relevance of hydration to each individual's clinical presentation, and above all, to be responsive to the wishes of the patient and the family'. Nevertheless they felt that 'In the absence of definitive research in this area, the balance of burdens and benefits of such treatment remains subjective. The prime goal of any treatment in terminal care should be the comfort of the patient. Decisions should be made on an individual basis, involving both patients and their carers wherever possible. Prolonging life in such circumstances is of secondary concern and i.v.fluids in this context may be futile.'[11]

However in a personal communication Ilora Finlay drew my attention to the value of subcutaneous fluids, and found them useful even in a patient's home.[13, 14].

A great deal of palliative care is undertaken by general physicians and consultant geriatricians in hospitals throughout the world. Their voice should be heard in the hydration debate. Yet in the corridors of power the tendency is to listen to the conservative voice of traditional palliative carers and to ignore those with opposing views. This will have devastating effects on the practice of medicine in the long term, for a policy of 'comfort care only' will shorten the lives of countless people who depend on artificial, or assisted nutrition and hydration for their survival.

4. Treatment of terminal agitation using sedation and hydration. A general physician's approach.

Terminal agitation has a variety of causes and is not confined to patients suffering from cancer. It may however, be more common in a hospice setting than elsewhere, although there appear to be no formal comparative studies to substantiate this possibility. It has been reported that up to 40% of hospice patients become agitated or restless in the last few days of life. This figure may be an underestimate for according to Bruera 22 to 24% of cases of agitated delirium are overlooked by physicians or nurses.[15] In my personal experience as a geriatrician, terminal agitation was unusual, but perhaps we overlooked some quietly agitated patients. Very few worrying examples come to mind. I recall one long stay patient who became agitated suddenly for no apparent reason; post mortem showed that he had suffered a pulmonary embolus. Another memorable elderly man with senile dementia refused to eat or drink and became inconsolable, worrying about hell and incidents that had occurred during his service in the Second World War. He required sedation with chlorpromazine, which proved somewhat ineffective.[16]

If the incidence of terminal agitation does indeed differ widely between health care settings, we need to look for an explanation. Given that the majority of people dying in a hospice suffer from cancer, the high incidence of terminal agitation may be due to some intrinsic factor related to disseminated cancer, or to toxicity due to opioids or other medication. Untreated dehydration could be an important factor since many hospice patients are known to die in a dehydrated state. Psychological factors such as the fear of impending death may be worse in a hospice than in places where some patients have the potential to recover. All these possibilities are worthy of study.

Terminal agitation may be due to severe anxiety or to any serious pathology that causes oxygen deficiency, low blood pressure, dehydration, sepsis, metabolic disturbance or damage to the brain. Patients with pre-existing mental illness may suffer a relapse associated with stress or the fear of impending death. Skilled psychiatric help should be sought under such circumstances. Clearly it is essential for the doctors to differentiate between reversible and irreversible causes of agitation for, as mentioned earlier, any state of agitation will prove terminal if treated by prolonged sedation without hydration.

Treatment will vary according to the circumstances and the views of the doctors concerned. If agitation is severe and the patient cannot swallow, sedation must be given by injection or infusion. Medication will vary. Some doctors will use drugs such as chlorpromazine or haloperidol, others will favour benzodiazepines of one sort or another. In a hospice setting, it is not unusual to sedate with injections of midazolam or methotrimeprazine given by continuous infusion using a syringe driver. The question of whether or not to give artificial hydration will arise if the patient becomes dehydrated or is at risk of dehydration. If there is any possibility that the agitation is due to a reversible factor, the maintenance of hydration is vital. When the underlying cause of agitation is irreversible, careful attention to hydration will prevent unnecessary discomfort and symptoms caused by dehydration.

Dr Maurice Jackson a Consultant Physician and Nephrologist working in an acute hospital unit in the UK has found a value for Diazemuls infusion in patients with terminal agitation, and in patients who require temporary sedation for conditions such as status epilepticus, acute psychosis, or violence during withdrawal from alcohol or drugs. In the short article that follows, Jackson outlines his experience in 50 patients. A longer article on this subject by Jackson was first published in Hospital Medicine in June 2000.[17] Most of Jackson's patients continued to eat or drink until shortly before they died, despite sedation with Diazemuls. Those who were unable to take oral fluids during sedation were given nasogastric tube feeding or intravenous fluids, so the problem of dehydration did not arise. Used in this way sedation did not appear to hasten death, but ensured that patients were calm and comfortable. Jackson now uses an infusion of Diazemuls in preference to treatment with midazolam or chlorpromazine in terminal agitation.

References

1. Bruera E. Franco JJ. Maltoni M. et al. Changing pattern of agitated impaired mental status in patients with advanced cancer: association with cognitive monitoring, hydration, and opioid rotation. *Journal of Pain and Symptom Management*, 1995; **10**:287-291.
2. Fainsinger RL. MacEachern T. Miller MJ. *et al*. The use of hypodermoclysis for rehydration in terminally ill cancer patients. Ibid. 1994; **9**: 298-302.
3. Proctoclysis for hydration of terminally ill cancer patients. Bruera E. Pruvost M. Schoeller T. et al. Ibid 1998; **15**: 216-219.
4. Sanders P. PEG. Complications in the community. *Geriatric Medicine*. 1996; **27**: 25-28.
5. CPR for people who are terminally ill. *European Journal of Palliative Care*. 1997; **4**(4); 125.

6. Sarhill N, Mahmoud FA, Christie R, Tahir A. Assessment of nutritional status and fluid deficits in advanced cancer. *Journal of Terminal Oncology,* 2003; **2:** 29-37.

7. Gillon R. Foreseeing is not necessarily the same as intending. *British Medical Journal.* 1999; **319**; 1431-2.

8. E David Cook. "Dying to die?" p.89 in Death without Dignity. Rutherford House Books. 1990.

9. Meystre CJN. Ahmedzai S. Burley NMJ. 'Terminally ill patients may want to live' (Letter). *British Medical Journal.* 1994; **309:** 409.

10. Fainsinger RL, Bruera E. When to treat dehydration in a terminally ill patient? *Support Cancer Care* 1997, Abstract Volume 5 (Issue 3); 205-211.

11. Dunphy K, Finlay I, Rathbone G, Gilbert J, Hicks F. Rehydration in palliative and terminal care: if not-why not? *Palliative Medicine* 1995; **9**: 221-228.

12. Ethical decision-making in palliative care: Artificial Hydration for people who are terminally ill. A paper prepared by joint working party between the National Council for Hospice and Specialist Palliative Care Services (NCHSPCS) and the Ethics Committee of the Association for Palliative Medicine of Great Britain and Ireland. *NCHSPCS*, London, July/August 1997.

13. Finlay I. Personal communication, November 1994.

14. McQuillan R, Finlay I. [Letter] Dehydration in dying patients. *Palliative Medicine* 1995; **9**: 341

15. Bruera E, Miller L, McCallion J et al. Cognitive failure in patients with terminal cancer: a prospective study. *Journal of Pain and Symptom Management* 1992; **7**: 192-195.

16. Craig GM, Unpublished personal observations from clinical practice.

17. Jackson MA. Peripheral infusion of Diazemuls. *Hospital Medicine* 2000; **61**: 412-416.

Chapter 12

Effective Treatment of Terminal Agitation Using Diazemuls

Maurice A Jackson, Consultant Physician and Nephrologist

Terminal agitation is a very unpleasant condition. It can be caused by many conditions, including metabolic encephalopathy which is usually due to electrolyte imbalance, nutritional disorders and sepsis. The condition is often complicated by problems such as fitting and alcohol withdrawal. In the hospice situation up to 40% of terminal patients develop restlessness and/or agitation in the last 24-48 hours and do not die peaceful deaths [1,2]. About 12% of dying patients develop jerking, or twitching.[2] In the acute general hospital, there will be many patients who are fitting as a result of cerebral tumours and acute metabolic disorders. Some patients will be withdrawing from alcohol and drugs. During the last 12 months at the Royal Wolverhampton Hospital, which has a catchment area of about 300,000 there were 1,543 deaths in the hospital.

After attempting to control severe status epilepticus in two patients who were dying from secondary malignant melanomas of the brain, I concluded that there must be a better and safer way of giving Diazemuls than just as repeat bolus injections. In both cases I had to give a bolus injection every 20-30 minutes to control the fits as the patients' conditions would lighten and they would start fitting; a further Diazemuls intravenous injection was required. The fitting would stop and the patients' conscious levels would fall, only for the whole sequence to be repeated about 30 minutes later.

Some pharmacological facts about Diazemuls.

- Diazemuls is licensed for sedation before procedures, premedication prior to anaesthesia, control of acute muscle spasm due to tetanus or poisoning, control of convulsions, status epilepticus and management of severe acute anxiety or agitation including delirium tremens [3]. The therapeutic action is rapid when given as a bolus intravenous injection. However, when the patient's condition is more chronic such as status epilepticus, alcohol or drug withdrawal or severe agitation, administration is more difficult.

- It was previously recommended that if the drug was to be given as an infusion that it should be mixed with 5% or 10% dextrose and then infused within 6 hours. The dosage of Diazemuls received over the 6 hours would be unpredictable because of strong adherence of the drug to polvinyl chloride (PVC) in the bag and the giving set [4,5,6].

- Diazemuls is legally classified as a controlled drug. Schedule 4, part 2. As such, the full controlled drug handling requirements associated with narcotic agents (controlled Drug Schedule 2) are avoided and nursing time reduced, which means that the logistical problems for nurses are much less than with narcotic agents.

- Diazemuls is an oil in water emulsion containing diazepam. This formulation reduces the risk of localized pain and thrombophlebitis [7]. Diazepam and its principal metabolite desmethyldiazepam are very potent anxiolytic agents .

Continuous infusion technique

- A peripheral cannula is inserted. Undiluted Diazemuls is drawn up into a 50 ml syringe (e.g. polyethylene Plastipac syringe from Becton Dickinson). Depending on the dosage required the syringe does not always require to be completely filled. A polyethylene, low sorbing extension set (IVAC G30303) is attached to the syringe and an IVAC 711 infusion pump is used. The Diazemols is infused according to Table 1, which shows recommended infusion rates, precautions and safety issues.
- The drug acts quickly and once the patient is stabilized it is rarely necessary to alter the dosage. We have not had any problems with superficial thrombophlebitis over and above those we would have anticipated with any normotonic infusion.
- The manufacturer's stability data shows that Diazemuls can be stored at 4 degrees centigrade in a polyethylene syringe for 28 days. This means that the syringes can be made up in the aseptic suite of the pharmacy department, and stored.

Table 1 Administration of Peripheral Diazemuls			
Detail	Preparation	Rate of infusion	Safety issues
Drug	Undiluted Diazemuls	**Most adults:** Commence at 2.5mg (0.5ml / hour). Increase in increments of 2.5mg/hour until control achieved	Infusion to be administered as sole drug through the intravenous cannula.
Syringe	50ml plastipak syringe (Becton Dickinson)[2]	Usual maintenance dose <7.4mg/hour[3]	If patient is not for terminal care, pulse oximetry should be used.
Giving Set	Low sorbing extension set (IVAC G30303)	Elderly: Commence at 1.25mg/hour (0.25ml/hour).	In the event of respiratory depression reverse with flumazenil (Anexate)
Pump	IVAC 711	Increase by increments of 1.25mg/hour until control achieved. _____ Nursing staff 'fine tune' the dosage.	Discuss with consultant if patient requiring > 20mg/hour

1. Diazemuls should not be mixed with any other solution except rarely with 10% or 20% Intralipid.
2. Change syringe and giving set every 24 hours.
3. Maximum therapeutic dosage so far recorded: 40mg/hour.

We have now successfully treated more than 50 patients with severe terminal agitation due to many causes including disseminated malignancy, cerebrovascular accidents, motor neurone disease, and metabolic disorders such as end stage hepatic and renal failure.

Results in patients with normal renal function. (Table 2)

The patients in Table 2 comprised the first 10 patients with normal renal function who were treated with the Diazemuls infusion. They had a number of conditions, which can result in patients becoming severely agitated when dying. Many were confused and frightened. The mean age of the patients was 70.8 years with a standard deviation of 7.8 years.

The mean dosage of Diazemuls required to control the symptoms of these patients was 7.4mg/hr, with a minimum dosage of 2mg/hr, and a maximum dosage of 17.5 mg/hr. The mean time that the patients required the Diazemuls infusion was 4.2 days, with two patients on the infusion for 9.0 days, and two patients on the infusion for one day only.

colspan table					

Table 2 Terminal agitation in patients with normal renal function

Shows the medical conditions of the patients and the dosage of Diazemuls required to keep them free from agitation

Patient number	Age	Medical conditions	Days on Diazemuls	Max.dosage of Diazemuls, mg/hour
1	69	Metastatic bladder & prostate cancer. Very agitatehr despite Diamorphine 80mg and Haloperidol 5mg. Diazemuls added.	7	5
2	63	Systemic sclerosis, rheumatoid arthritis. pseudomembranous colitis, bleeding leg ulcers, ischaemic heart disease, polycystic kidneys and status epilepticus.	6	15
3	77	Pneumonia/pleurisy, severe COPD, LVF * not responding to therapy. Very agitated despite diamorphine for 8 days. Diamorphine stopped, Diazemuls started.	1	5
4	78	Disseminated cancer of the stomach, unable to eat or 9 5mg/hr drink. Very distressed	9	5
5	57	Alcoholic liver disease. hepatic encephalopathyhr pseudobulbar palsy, osteomyelytis, staphylococcus aureus septicaemia.	4	10
6	67	Wegener's Granulomatosis, MRSA infection fo large lung granuloma despite partial lobectomy no response to treatment.	9	5
7	84	Dense right hemiparesis, very agitated, history of alcohol excess.	5	17.5
8	73	Cancer of lung, metastases in bone. Very agitater despite diamorphine and haloperidol.	3	4.5
9	71	Motor neurone disease, continuously chokinhr Unable to sleep.	1	2
10	69	Respiratory failure due to pulmonary fibrosis Cheyne Stokes respiration. Very agitated despite Diamorphine. Diamorphine stopped. Diazumols alone- dramatic improvement.	3	5

Note. COPD = chronic obstructive pulmonary disease. LVF = left ventricular failure.

Table reprinted from Hospital Medicine 2000; 61: p 213 with the Editor's kind permission.

It can be seen from Table 2 that three of the patients had disseminated malignancy. The majority of patients on the diazemuls regimen continue to take food and fluid until shortly before death. If they are unable to take nutrients and fluid then a nasogastric tube feed is started. If the patient is unable to tolerate a nasogastric tube or if like patient 4 there is a total blockage of the stomach or oesophagus then intravenous fluids are given to prevent dehydration. Patients 1 and 8 became very agitated despite diamorphine and haloperidol, but rapidly improved when the Diazemuls infusion was added. The severely agitated symptoms of patients 3 and 10 were not controlled with diamorphine but there was a dramatic improvement when the diamorphine was stopped and Diazemuls was started. Patient 2 had systemic sclerosis, and developed intractable fits at a time when it had already been decided that further treatment would be inappropriate. Despite weighing less than 60 kg, this patient required 15mg/hr of Diazemuls to control her symptoms and fits.

Patient 7 required 17.5 mg Diazemuls per hour. This patient had a massive cerebral infarct affecting his dominant side. He was extremely agitated. A safe environment could not be maintained because the patient was constantly trying to get out of bed. He continuously tried to remove his catheter. The patient had a very long history of alcohol excess. Once stable on 17.5 mg/hr of Diazemuls, this patient remained comfortable. Any attempt to lower the dosage caused his problems to recur. Patient 5 also had a long history of alcohol excess and required 10mg/hr to control symptoms.

Patient 9 had very severe motor neurone disease and was choking on her own secretions. She was terrified of choking and had been unable to sleep for a number of days. After full discussion with the patient and her family, she was started on the Diazemuls infusion. She fell asleep about two hours later and had a very comfortable night. She died peacefully the following day.

Four patients in this group were on diamorphine and haloperidol. Two of the patients no longer required these drugs when Diazemuls was started. The dosage of haloperidol and diamorphine remained constant in the other two patients.

Most of the patients continued to eat and drink until shortly before they died. If a patient was not able to take oral fluids, a nasogastric tube feed was instituted. All drugs, except those for symptomatic benefit, were stopped at the time of starting the infusion of Diazemuls, if the patients were being treated for terminal agitation.

It is imperative to ensure that sedation does not mask pain, and to treat pain effectively if it is present.

Results in 22 patients with terminal renal failure

In a study of chronic haemodialysis patients where haemodialysis was withdrawn due to other severe medical conditions or very poor quality of life, the mean time from withdrawal of dialysis to death was 7.2 (SE+1.6) days with a range of 2.0 to 22.0 days. In all patients, the mean length of time on the Diazemuls infusion was 3.3 (SE+0.6) days with a maximum of 14.0 days and a minimum of 6.0 hours. The overall mean dose was 4.3 (SE+0.7) mg/hr with a maximum of 10.0 mg/hr and a minimum of 1.0 mg/hr. Eight of the 22 patients required 2.5 mg/hr.

The mean age of the renal failure patients treated with the Diazemuls infusion was 74.4 years with a standard deviation of 7.8. There was no significant difference in the ages of patients with normal and abnormal renal function or in the number of days they were on the infusion. The renal failure patients required a slightly lower dose of Diazemuls than the patients with normal renal function (mean dosage Diazemuls 7.4mg/hr SD 5.09. P=0.011).

Results in non-terminal patients who recovered

The patients who were not being treated for terminal agitation were much younger (mean age 36.4 years, SD+14.0), but there was no significant difference in the number of days on the infusion (mean 2.3 days, SD+1.6), however, the dosage of Diazemuls required was much greater (19.3 mg/hr, SD+ 26.1). These patients were being treated for status epilepticus, alcohol and drug withdrawal, and control of violence.

In one patient who was very agitated at night, but not during the day, the infusion rate was increased each night (eg. 2.5 mg/hr during the day and 10.0 mg/hr during the night). It was rarely necessary to increase the dose of Diazemuls after control of symptoms was obtained.

Conclusions

Those patients who were terminally agitated all died comfortable, non-agitated deaths. The treatment does not appear to hasten death. We suspect that those patients who were previously treated with diamorphine and whose symptoms were not properly controlled lived longer on the Diazemuls infusion than if they had remained on the narcotic agents. The patient, relatives, and nurses were much less stressed when the patient's symptoms were properly controlled.

The continuous infusion of Diazemuls by our method has proved effective in our patients. The patients are much more comfortable and are no longer agitated. The treatment does not appear to hasten death. Previously we have used infusions of midazolam and chlorpromazine to treat this group of patients but these drugs were very poor at controlling the patient's symptoms of agitation and were therefore largely discontinued.

There has been a lot of recent concern with the way that doctors manage dying patients and the use of narcotic agents in these patients [10,11]. Treatment with Diazemuls appears to be an appropriate, very effective, simple and inexpensive way of looking after patients who are otherwise going to die an unpleasant death with terminal agitation.

References

1. Lichter I, Hunt E . The last 48 hours of life. *Journal of Palliative Care*. 1990; **6(4)**: 4-8.
2. Saunders C. Pain and impending death. In: Wall PD, Melzack R, eds. Textbook of Pain, 2nd edn. Churchill Livingstone, Edinburgh: 1989; p.624-631.
3. ABPI Compendium of Data Sheets and Summaries of Product Characteristics 1998-1999, Datapharm Publications Limited, London, 1998.

4. Martens HJ, De Goede PN, Van Loienen AC. Sorption of various drugs in polyvinyl chloride, glass, and polyethylene-lined infusion containers. *American Journal of Hospital Pharmacy.* 1990; **47**: 369- 373.
5. Winsnes M, Jeppsson R, Sjoberg B. Diazepam adsorption to infusion sets and plastic syringes. *Acta Anaesthesiologica Scandinavica.* 1981; **25**: 93-96
6. Hancock BG, Black DB. Effect of a polyethylene-lined administration set on the availability of diazepam injection. *American Journal of Hospital Pharmacy.* 1985; **42**: 2335-2339
7. Von Dardel O, Mebius C, Mossberg T, Svensson B. Fat emulsion as a vehicle for diazepam. A study of 9492 patients. *British Journal of Anaesthesia.* 1983; **55**: 41-47
8. Jack ML, Colburn WA. Pharmacokinetic model for diazepam and its major metabolite desmethyldiazepam following diazepam administration. *Journal of Pharmaceutical Science.* 1983; **72**: 1318-1323
9. Greenblatt DJ, Divoll MK, Soong MH, Boxenbaum HG, Harmatz JS, Shader RI. Desmethyldiazepam Pharmacokinetics: studies following intravenous and oral LDesmethyldiazepam, oral clorazepate, and intravenous diazepam. *Journal of Clinical Pharmacology.* 1988; **28**: 853-859
10. Gillon R. When doctors might kill their patients. *British Medical Journal.* 1999; **318**:1431-1432
11. Doyal L. The moral character of clinicians or the best interests of patient? *British Medical Journal.* 1999; **318**:1432-1433.

Chapter 13

Legal Issues

Is Sedation Without Hydration or Nourishment in Terminal Care Lawful?

Author Gillian Craig
**This paper was first published in the Medico Legal Journal in 1994;
62:198-201. It is reprinted with permission.**

There are occasions in palliative medicine, when the responsible doctor considers it necessary to use sedation to the point where the patient becomes so drowsy that he/she is unable to eat or drink in the normal way. It is not unknown for such sedation to be continued for as long as seven days before the patient finally dies. Under such circumstances the patient will become fatally dehydrated unless some measures are taken to prevent this, yet such measures may not be taken. Non intervention is on occasions a deliberate and firmly held policy that is maintained by the responsible medical team despite the concerns expressed by others. This situation is dangerous, medically, ethically and legally for reasons that have been argued in a recent article in the Journal of Medical Ethics.[1] Great distress can be caused to dissenting relatives, and there is at present no formal mediation procedure to which they can resort.

Legal aspects have been touched on in the initial article,[1] and were further discussed in a helpful editorial by Dr R. Gillon,[2] but further debate is needed within the legal profession, on the legality of withholding life-prolonging treatment, or fluids and nutrition in the dying. This has not yet been specifically tested in the courts of the United Kingdom, although the situation as it relates to patients with a persistent vegetative state (pvs) has been clarified. In the case of patients with pvs the Law Lords ruling in the case of Airedale and NHS Trust v Bland, was that artificial feeding through a naso-gastric tube was a form of life support which could be discontinued if treatment was futile and no longer in the best interests of the patient. The judgement was swayed by the patient's irreversible brain damage and the lack of awareness, and by the fact that he was unable to swallow as a result of this. Considerable safeguards were devised to protect patients with pvs from premature withdrawal of sustenance. No such safeguards exist for patients who are thought to be terminally ill.

Unlike patients with pvs, those with an illness that is believed by the doctor to be terminal may be alert and compos mentis until they are rendered sleepy or comatose by sedation. This can be initiated on the word of one doctor. Some may have their swallowing impaired by disease, others will have been able to eat or drink normally until sedated. Thereafter they will be rendered incapable of maintaining their own nutrition and hydration, and will inevitably die within about seven days unless steps are taken to hydrate them by artificial means.

Sedation of the sort that is discussed in this paper is used in terminal care in situations where patient management is proving extremely difficult. The problem may be one of intractable pain, of acute shortness of breath, or of psychological distress. Psychological distress may be due to an underlying psychiatric disorder, to overwhelming anxiety about impending death, or to an acute confusional state, due perhaps to an infection. Many of these factors are potentially treatable. To opt for sedation, without hydration, will mean that some patients will die unnecessarily early. Doctors are not renowned for their accuracy in predicting how long a patient has to live. One study found them to be accurate to within a month only 16% of the time. Some patients who are considered to be terminally ill by one doctor, are cured by another. It is also recognised that there is a risk of inappropriate sedation, for reasons related to the distress of the carers, rather than of the patient. Faced with this information there is clearly a need to safeguard the interests of the patient whenever a regime of sedation without hydration is thought to be necessary. I would suggest that such patients should be reviewed by at least one, and preferably two consultants, one of whom should be practising in an appropriate acute specialty.

Intractable pain should rarely be a problem with skilled management and appropriate referral in cases of difficulty. There is no place for trying to solve the problem by lethal injections, however desperate the situation and, in my view, Dr Cox was rightly convicted of attempted murder in a recent case. It was suggested in correspondence in the British Medical Journal that Dr Cox could have avoided this outcome by using continuous intravenous or subcutaneous midazolam.

There is a vogue at present for treating severe pain with high doses of pain killers, and as a last resort, induction of sleep with midazolam. The advent of syringe drivers means that this treatment can now be given in the patient's home at the instigation of their general practitioner. Midazolam is a benzodiazepine, of the same family of drugs as Valium and temazepam. It is licensed in the United Kingdom for short term use, as an intravenous sedative during minor medical procedures, such as endoscopy, as an intramuscular premedication for surgery, and as an intravenous agent for induction- i.e. initiation of anaesthesia in certain patients. The data sheet does not indicate that it has been authorised for continuous use over a matter of days, and such use may be beyond the bounds of the product licence. Other drugs such as methotrimeprazine, a sedative allied to chlorpromazine, are given subcutaneously by continuous infusion in some cases where psychological distress is troublesome. Whatever drug regime is used for sedation, the patient will be at risk of dehydration unless steps are taken to prevent this. Such active intervention goes against hospice philosophy.[1]

The magnitude of this problem needs to be assessed by a national survey of the use of midazolam and other sedatives in terminal care. We need to know the indication for use, the duration of use, and the final outcome. The views of close relatives should be obtained. Some will be content with management, others will experience long term distress. Such a study would be facilitated if all deaths involving the use of parenteral sedation were to be referred to the coroner routinely. It is widely recognised that some essential medical interventions may inadvertently shorten life, and if this occurs in good faith, the doctor is rarely considered to be to blame. This principle of double effect is stated in one text book as follows- "A good objective may be performed despite the fact that the objective can only be achieved at the expense of a coincidental harmful effect." [3] This principle is open to abuse, and could be quoted in the defence of medical practitioners whose standards of care and intentions are open to question. The example usually given is that of pain control. High doses of opiates for example may increase the risk of death from respiratory depression and retained secretion. Drugs such as nalorphine antagonise the pain relief, so side effects may be unavoidable. However as Lord Edmund Davies commented "Killing both pain and patient may be good morals but it is far from certain that it is good law." [3] It is far from certain that it is good medicine either. Much of the skill of modern medicine involves the recognition and avoidance of potential side effects in order to achieve useful benefits for the patient. Medicine at its best is a sophisticated art. The law as it is applied to medicine should demand a high standard of practice.

Where the side effects of a given treatment such as sedation are predictable, lethal, and easily overcome by simple measures such as intravenous fluids to prevent dehydration, failure to use such measures could be regarded as negligence and warrants a conviction for manslaughter. These days the use of intravenous fluids cannot be regarded as an extraordinary measure. It is not however a measure that can be continued for more than a week or so, but if the patient is truly terminally ill, death from natural causes will intervene before problems with drip maintenance arise. There are other routes by which fluids can be given if need be.

The House of Lords Select Committee on Medical Ethics considered the question of treatment-limiting decisions and agreed that there is a point at which the duty to try to save the patient's life is exhausted, and at which continued treatment may be inappropriate. Such a point must be identified in the light of each patient's individual condition and circumstances. The committee were unable to reach agreement on the question of whether nutrition and hydration, even when given by invasive methods, may ever be regarded as treatment, which in certain circumstances it may be inappropriate to initiate or continue. In the case of a patient with pvs it was hoped that the patient would succumb to pneumonia before the question of withdrawing hydration or nutrition arose.[4] One useful concept voiced by the committee was that a decision to limit treatment may depend on the balance between the burdens which the treatment will impose, and the benefits it is likely to produce. They made it clear that it should be unnecessary to consider the withdrawal (or non-introduction) of nutrition and hydration, except in circumstances where its administration is in itself burdensome to the patient.[4]

The British Medical Association, quoted by Dr Gillon, advise that "although doctors should not give treatment simply because it is available, in cases of doubt about the best interests of the patient the presumption should be in favour of prolonging life." [2]

Thus the philosophy and practice and non-intervention in matters of hydration, advocated by some specialists in palliative medicine, and taught by them to trainee general practitioners cannot be accepted uncritically and are being questioned. [1] The debate will no doubt continue but I hope that medical practice will change. Sooner or later the legality of sedation without hydration or nutrition in the dying must be tested in the courts.

References

1. Craig GM. On withholding nutrition and hydration in the terminally ill: has palliative medicine gone too far? *Journal of Medical Ethics* 1994; 20:139-143.
2. Gillon R. Editorial. Palliative care ethics: non-provision of artificial nutrition and hydration to terminally ill sedated patients. *Journal of Medical Ethics.* 1994; 20: 131-132,187.
3. "Euthanasia" p 230-249 in Law and Medical Ethics. Mason JK and McCall Smith RA. London, *Butterworths* 1987.
4. House of Lords Select Committee on Medical Ethics. Report. Paragraphs 251-257. Treatment-limiting decisions. London. *HMSO* 1994.

ON DOUBLE EFFECT AND OTHER LEGAL ISSUES

© *Craig 2003*

My aim in this paper is to continue the discussion on double effect, taking as the starting point my article in the Medico-Legal Journal of 1994.[1] The question for debate remains – 'Is sedation without hydration or nourishment in terminal care lawful?' Surprising though it may seem, despite the passage of time, this important matter has not yet been settled in the courts in the United Kingdom. Some may share the view of Ashby and Stoffell who noted in 1995 that the lack of case law on the issue of abatement of artificial hydration and nutrition in dying persons could be 'because no court has been asked specifically to consider it. This seems to indicate that in practice it has not been seen to be an issue that requires legal judgement'.[2] I hope to persuade my readers that this is an important and complex medico-legal issue that deserves serious attention from the legal profession. Some lawyers are now showing an interest in the problem, but when a potential test case has been identified it requires superhuman effort to get it to a court. Access to justice is not easy for members of the public, and few have the emotional stamina or financial resources to stay the course. In addition lawyers and judges are not trained in medicine and rely heavily on the views of the medical profession who tend to protect their colleagues.

In law, according to Fletcher, a doctor may be criminally liable either for intentionally taking life, or for omitting to act and thus permitting death to occur. Acting intentionally to cause death is unconditionally prohibited. Permitting a patient to die functions as an omission in legal analysis.[3] Doctors are legally responsible for their acts and their omissions. For all the above reasons it can be argued that to end a person's life intentionally by withholding hydration is illegal. An exception to this has been made in the UK with respect to patients in a permanent vegetative state, but at present all such cases have to go through the courts.

The legal position with regard to a sedated and terminally ill patient is not straightforward. A respected lawyer, working with the Official Solicitor, writing to me in 1994 said, 'There is no doubt in my mind that in the present state of the law it would not be lawful to withdraw artificial feeding and hydration from a terminally ill sedated patient, unless it could be shown that either the patient was in a persistent vegetative state, or that possibly a valid advance directive had been signed'.[4]

Macleod, in an article on the management of delirium in hospice practice said, 'To anaesthetise in the absence of a life support system is generally considered to be legally unacceptable and a form of euthanasia'.[5] The same could be said of prolonged sedation without hydration. Midazolam, one of the drugs commonly used for sedation in the dying, is licensed as an anaesthetic induction agent for short-term use. It was never intended to be used for days on end without hydration. However those responsible for post-marketing drug evaluation at the Department of Health while agreeing that the use of medicines as licensed is desirable, consider it important to recognise that doctors may sometimes need to use medicines outside the conditions specified in the licence and are entitled to do so if they see fit. When I raised this issue with them in 1995 my correspondent felt that the issue of fluid replacement for patients who are terminally ill and require sedation relates to the practice of medicine in terminal care rather than the intrinsic safety of the relevant medicines. Since the Committee on Safety of Medicines has no remit to advise doctors on how to practice medicine, it was considered inappropriate for them to take any action on this issue.[6]

A retired Consultant in Palliative Medicine writing in 1997 told me, 'An enquiry into the use of sedation is overdue. Powerful agents such as methotrimeprazine and midazolam are being administered widely by subcutaneous continuous infusion in the terminal phase in hospices to an extent of which the profession at large may not be aware'.[7] It has now been acknowledged by the Royal College of Physicians that this practice is 'very common'.[8]

Sadly it is a fact that desperately difficult situations do arise from time to time in the care of the dying. There are occasions when patients are delirious or have pain that is difficult to control. Such cases tax the skills of palliative carers and make some sedation essential. However it does not necessarily follow that hydration should be withheld once the crisis has been controlled.

An honest debate of the ethical issues and very careful review of the clinical situation is essential.

Proportionality comes into the equation. The benefit to be gained by intervention should be proportional to the risks and burdens of intervention and vice versa. Thus when a person's life expectancy is only one or two weeks, invasive techniques for the maintenance of hydration and nutrition such as a gastrostomy, would be considered inappropriate, whereas simpler measures such as a naso-gastric tube or subcutaneous fluids could be justified on many grounds.

It is extremely dangerous to label a person terminally ill and in imminent danger of death, and then to treat - and continue to treat - in such a way that death becomes inevitable. Such management should not be tolerated. Imminent death must surely mean that the patient is expected to die of his or her condition within a matter of days. To say that death is imminent and then starve the patient for weeks until they die is a cynical and self-fulfilling prophecy unworthy of a doctor. A member of the public who behaved in this way would be guilty of a criminal offence and jailed. In Australia a person died having followed the instructions of a cult leader who recommended a long period of abstinence from food and water for spiritual enlightenment. The man responsible for the fast was charged with manslaughter.[9] Why should a doctor who withholds hydration and food from a patient be treated any differently?

When the benefit is life itself, and the prevention of symptoms due to dehydration doctors should think very carefully indeed before withholding hydration. If life itself no longer appears to be a benefit, we enter dangerous territory. Some people who advocate euthanasia would like to be able to solve the problem with a lethal injection. Others, including the majority of palliative care specialists would strive to control pain and other symptoms until the patient died. Current professional guidelines should ensure that hydration is kept under constant review and used appropriately in dying patients.[10] Sedation without hydration may be appropriate on rare occasions but only if this regime can be justified on medical, ethical and legal grounds. A patient who is hydrated but not fed for weeks on end will die just as surely as a person who is sedated and dehydrated for days, or given a lethal injection. The crucial issue in law is the doctor's intent. It is surely time for the legal profession to ensure that all patients, including those who are thought to be dying, have protection under the law.

The doctrine of double effect.

The doctrine of double effect remains an important defence for doctors who have to use powerful drugs to control pain or mental distress in the dying. It has been described by one lawyer, somewhat cynically, as 'the get out of jail free card'.[11] In essence it states that 'A good objective may be performed despite the fact that the objective can only be achieved at the expense of a coincidental harmful effect'. In palliative care the good effect intended is usually pain relief, the bad effect may be that life is shortened. Unfortunately the principle is open to abuse and can become a smokescreen for euthanasia.

According to Price the doctrine of double effect has four conditions to be satisfied- viz.

- The action itself (divorced from its consequences) must not be inherently morally wrong.
- The intention must be solely to produce the good effect.
- The good effect must not be achieved through the means of the bad effect (causally speaking).
- There must be a favourable balance between the good and the bad effects of the action.[12]

Potentially lethal palliation should not be considered unless other safer forms of treatment have been tried without success, and all other avenues have been exhausted. There must be a proportionately grave reason for the action taken. The good effect, e.g. pain relief, must be sufficiently worthwhile to justify the bad effect such as shortening life. The question of justification is complex, for as Price notes- 'justification is a composite of a number of (objective) factors, and not purely dictated by reference to the state of mind of the actor.' [12] Where the risk of shortening life is considerable, some take the view that potentially lethal palliation should only be permissible in cases of terminal illness.[13] Others however would disagree.

With respect to the use of sedation without hydration, I take the view that where the side effects of a given treatment such as sedation are predictable, lethal, and easily overcome by simple measures such as the use of intravenous or subcutaneous fluids to prevent dehydration, failure to use such measures could be considered negligent.[1] Doctors when giving potentially lethal palliation, as with any dangerous procedure, should ask themselves whether they can avoid unintended and potentially lethal side effects such as dehydration or respiratory depression. If they can prevent side effects, but choose not to do so, their intention may not be honourable. For the doctrine of double effect to be a valid defence, the doctor's primary intention should be to relieve pain or mental distress. Intentional killing is unlawful. If, despite having achieved the primary aim, medication is continued until the patient becomes fatally dehydrated the doctor's intentions should be called into question.

Two editorials in the British Medical Journal are of interest.[14] They were written by medical ethicists, both of whom are, or were, members of the Medical Ethics Committee of the British Medical Association. They were commenting on the acquittal of a doctor who had given a dying patient a lethal dose of diamorphine. Raanon Gillon, said, 'If, despite relieving the pain and distress, one goes on giving more heroin until the patient does die... then clearly one not only foresees the patient's death - one intends it.' Len Doyal was more provocative and took the view that non-treatment decisions, or potentially lethal palliation could be in the patient's best interest. He argued, 'It is time we stopped avoiding real debate on the possible legalisation of active euthanasia by pretending that the double effect argument will somehow resolve it for us. It will not'. Doyal appears to advocate involuntary euthanasia under circumstances that are not covered by 'double effect'. For example he hints that death might be desirable for an elderly man, temporally mentally incapacitated by treatable illness, whose quality of life is poor because of loneliness, poverty and failing eyesight.[14] When a medical ethicist argues thus we are on a very slippery slope indeed. Clearly rigorous interpretation of the law is vital if patients are to be protected from those who seek to end their lives.

The criminal law in a nutshell states that intentional killing is murder, reckless killing is manslaughter, negligence is manslaughter, and death is sometimes accidental.

In criminal law, if death is foreseen as virtually certain to occur, and death does occur, that death is murder. In a medical context there is a less stringent approach, and intention is narrowly defined as purpose or desire, according to Penney Lewis, lecturer in medical law at the Institute of Law and Medical Ethics at King's College, London. Speaking on double effect at the Royal College of Physicians in 1997 Lewis told doctors that a concealed defence is not a good idea, for it has the disadvantage of uncertainty and unpredictability. Lewis discussed three possible approaches to legislation in the future, any of which, she thought, would be better than the current ad hoc approach in the UK-

- *The defence of necessity*. This is the argument that the doctor had a conflict of duties and could not end suffering without ending life. This would be an extremely rare situation in the hands of a skilled doctor. However in the Netherlands, 'necessity' was the argument that led to euthanasia becoming de facto lawful. This outcome might be avoided in the UK by restricting the defence of necessity to cases where the doctor's purpose is not to cause death. At present under English law duress and necessity are rarely permitted as defences to murder, according to Price.[12]
- *A specific statutory defence applying only to palliative care relief could be built into the law of murder*. Legislation to this effect has been passed in South Australia (Act No 26 of 1995). Life-shortening treatment is now permissible if given with the intention of relieving pain or distress in terminal illness, with the patient's consent. It must be administered in good faith and in accordance with professional standards of palliative care.[12]
- *Evaluation and justification of the doctor's action could be built into part 2 of the criminal law relating to intent*. This proposal, (coming from Finnis of Oxford University) would include within the law of murder doing without lawful justification or excuse, an act which one is sure would kill. Thus within the law of murder one could assess whether or not there was lawful justification or excuse.

It remains to be seen whether any changes will be made to the law.

A theological comment

An Anglican Bishop, John Austin Baker made the following helpful comments on double effect in a letter to me – 'Double effect is still the basic approach of, for example, the Catholic Church, and widely used by other Christians. And of course, we all know there are cases where it is entirely relevant. But, as you say, it can be abused. It seems to me that progress could be made by unpacking the ideas a bit.

'If we assume that the medical treatment envisaged should be that best given for medical reasons, even though life may be thereby shortened, what are the objectives the doctor should be trying to achieve? In the very simple cases usually quoted, the overriding objective is to relieve intolerable pain. So pain relief is a legitimate medical objective. If one is working in a hospice context, one might talk of making the patient comfortable, so that his/her last days or hours may be ones of dignity, with the ability to receive and give affection to others, to be clear headed enough to say what one wants to say, and so forth. It follows that whatever palliative care is provided should seek to maximise these things as far as may be. Clearly decisions have to be made case by case. But it would seem to an observer such as myself, that if the withdrawal of nourishment or hydration increased distress or discomfort, that would be a reason for not doing that- not just an ethical but a medical reason. To insist on doing it would mean that the only reason for the action was to shorten life, and double effect would not apply.'

The Bishop added, 'In the end it comes down to this: does such withdrawal, particularly of hydration (where hydration is practicable) increase suffering? As you say yourself, we need more unbiased research to establish the answer. The commonsense view of lay people who have been seriously ill, is that it would'.[15]

Intention, purpose and side effects

Legal minds are now addressing the concept of 'primary purpose' and 'secondary purposes.' Some, for example Lord Donaldson, as quoted by Price are inclined to view secondary consequences (such as death) arising from medical treatment decisions made in the patient's best interest, as mere side effects.[16] Others argue that secondary purposes cannot be ignored. Price quotes Clarkson and Keating who said 'A defendant can have two or more purposes in acting. Both purposes are intended'.[17] 'How, if there was a secondary purpose in the physician's mind that the patient should die as a result of his actions, could the law ignore this?' asks Price. How indeed! Yet the crucial question as to why palliative carers continue to give sedation and often fail to treat consequent dehydration, with lethal consequences, has yet to be addressed in a court of law. Yet as Price notes it would in general be feasible to decide 'whether an omission was culpable', the central issue being 'the duties of the doctor founded on the interests and rights of the patient'.[12]

Sedation without hydration

Clearly the legal situation with regard to sedation without hydration is complex, for it involves an act and an omission. The initial purpose of the act of sedation may be to relieve distress, or to prevent harm to the patient or a third party, if the patient is violent or noisy, for example. Sometimes a patient is sedated for the benefit of carers who cannot stand the situation. Whatever the reason the patient is likely to become dehydrated unless steps are taken to prevent this.

Let us assume that the primary reason, intent or purpose for sedation is reasonable and good. What reason might a doctor have for refusing to prevent death from dehydration? What secondary purposes might there be for inaction? Well the doctor might consider that the underlying cause of the patient's distress was irreversible, and difficult to control, so that sedation would need to be continued for a long time, possibly indefinitely. In that case it might be reasonable not to prolong life artificially in a patient whose life expectancy was short. However if the distress was relieved by sedation, what reason might there be for failing to support life by simple measures? (See Table 1)

Table 1 Factors that might influence the doctor to withold treatment-
- A sense of futility, a generally hopeless situation.
- A desire not to disturb the patient's acceptance of death.
- A desire to get it over, not to prolong dying.
- A competent patient's informed and expressed views.
- A patient's non-specific dislike of medical intervention.
- A desire not to cause the patient distress.
- Technically impossible to hydrate or feed.
- Inadequate resources available.
- Opportunity costs. Bed needed for someone else.
- Death inevitable and imminent with or without hydration.
- Compassion- but it should be 'correct compassion.' Always remember that compassion need not and must not kill.
- The thought that the patient would be better off dead. This may be masked by the phrase 'in the patient's best interest.'
- A relative's request to stop treatment.
- A valid advance directive, or decision by legal proxy prohibiting intervention.

Some of the reasons shown in Table 1 are valid and lawful, others are not. Once in a while withholding hydration or nutrition will amount to criminal negligence or murder. Clearly there is considerable scope for legal discussion to founder in semantic arguments about foresight, intention, primary and secondary purposes and so on. The key point to remember is that water is essential for life. If hydration is withheld the patient will die. If hydration can be provided, and life supported without undue discomfort or risk to the patient, a doctor's reason for withholding it should be subjected to close scrutiny. It is not sufficient to say vaguely that you are removing a burden or that treatment is not benefiting the patient. If the intention or purpose (be it primary or secondary) of withholding hydration is to shorten life, the doctor should be culpable in law, unless there is valid justification for inaction.

If death is clearly seen as an inevitable consequence of a doctor's action or inaction, a doctor may not be blameless in law, for as Price noted 'in very many scenarios a realisation that consequences will ensue from one's actions *is* tantamount to intention in law.'[12]

The neglect factor

It is now recognised in legal circles that death can be due to natural causes contributed to by neglect. Such a verdict is the preferred modern terminology for a verdict of 'lack of care' in a coroner's court. Clues as to current legal thinking in the UK on the subject of neglect can be found in the judgement in the Court of Appeal in the Touche case [18] and in another important negligence case (R v North Humberside ex parte Jamieson.) [19]

The Touche case was brought by the widower of a woman who died of a cerebral haemorrhage following a Caesarian section. It was alleged that monitoring of her blood pressure had been inadequate, and that this had contributed to her death. The widower had considerable difficulty persuading the coroner to hold an inquest and took his fight to the High Court. The coroner appealed against a decision by a Divisional Court that an inquest should be held. In his Appeal Court judgement in March 2001, Lord Justice Simon Brown referred to conclusions drawn from another case, that of R v North Humberside ex parte Jamieson,[20] which he described as 'a landmark decision in coronial law given in the context of a prisoner who had hanged himself in a prison hospital cell.' Lord Justice Brown quoted some conclusions about neglect, as taken from the Jamieson case by Mr Burnett QC acting for the Appellant in Touche. They are broad conclusions that have considerable general medico-legal relevance - (see Table 2)

Table 2. Medico-legal criteria for neglect.

1. 'self-neglect is a gross failure to take adequate nourishment of liquid or to obtain basic medical attention or adequate shelter or warmth;
2. 'neglect is the obverse of self-neglect;
3. 'neglect means a gross failure to provide basic medical attention for someone in a depenedent position (for example because of illness) who cannot provide it for himself;
4. ' the need for basic medical attention must be obvious;
5. 'the crucial consideration is what the condition of the dependent person appeared to be;
6. 'neglect can rarely if ever be an appropriate verdict on its own but it may be factually accurate to say that it contributed to death;
7. 'neither neglect nor self-neglect should ever form part of a verdict unless a clear and direct causal connection is established between the conduct so described and the cause of death.'[21]

In the opinion of Lord Justice Brown, neglect does not have to involve a gross failure to supply an obvious basic need in order to be significant. Lesser degrees of neglect may also be significant. In the Touche case the neglect consisted of failure to monitor the patient's blood pressure for a two and a half hour period during the critical post-operative phase after a Caesarian section, with the result that there was some delay in detecting a rise in blood pressure, the possible consequence being that a fatal cerebral haemorrhage was not prevented. The Appeal Court directed that an inquest should be held. In due course an inquest was held, and in March 2002 the jury decided unanimously that Mrs Laura Touche had died of natural causes contributed to by neglect.[22]

The wider implications of Touche

Let us now compare the situation of the late Mrs Touche with that of a terminally ill sedated patient who is deprived of fluids and nourishment for days on end, with the consequence that gross dehydration develops. The question at issue is, does the failure to provide fluid by artificial or assisted means amount to gross failure to meet an obvious basic need? It is surely time to settle this matter in court, given the fact that the use of sedation is 'very common' in the last days of life.[8]

Section 8 (3) of the Coroner's Act of 1988 requires that an inquest must be held with a jury 'if it appears to the coroner…that death occurred in circumstances the continuance or possible recurrence of which is prejudicial to the health or safety of the public or any section of the public.' It could be said that the practice of sedation without hydration is prejudicial to the health and safety of terminally ill patients and may shorten their lives.

The recognition that death can be due to natural causes contributed to by neglect is helpful, for it is rarely possible to be absolutely certain of the cause of death in a patient with gross dehydration and serious pathology such as widespread cancer. However *gross dehydration should not be ignored by the legal profession, for it is not irrelevant. It could in some cases be the final cause of death.* The facts should be ascertained carefully to see whether dehydration appears to be a significant factor contributing to death. As Lord Justice Brown noted in the case of McGhee v National Coal Board there may be factors (in a death) "that may well be secondary but are not self-evidently irrelevant."[23] In the course of that case Lord Justice Brown concluded, "It seems to me necessary to recognise that cases may well arise in which human fault can and properly should be found to turn what would otherwise be a natural death into an unnatural one, and one into which therefore an inquest should be held."[24]

Predominantly therapeutic acts

There is a growing recognition by lawyers that therapeutic omissions can be just as lethal as acts. When the euthanasia working group chaired by Judge Stephen Tumim published their position statement on medical treatment at the end of life in the spring of 2000 they introduced the phrase 'predominantly therapeutic acts' to encompass decisions that involve omissions such as withholding and withdrawing futile or burdensome treatment, with the foreseen but unintended consequence that life may be shortened [25]. Thus we are left with the strange situation that acts such as giving a lethal injection are considered unlawful, but predominantly therapeutic acts, as defined above are condoned by many people.

Controversial guidance has been produced by the British Medical Association on the subject of withholding and withdrawing life-prolonging medical treatment. This guidance does not address the care of the dying in any depth, but concentrates on decisions to withhold or withdraw treatment from patients who could live for weeks, months or possibly years if treatment such as artificial hydration and nutrition was provided. The BMA use a very narrow definition of basic care and limit this to 'those procedures essential to keep an individual comfortable.' These include the provision of warmth, shelter, pain relief, management of distressing symptoms, hygiene measures, and the offer of oral nutrition and hydration.[26] The provision of artificial or assisted hydration and nutrition is not considered to be basic care by the BMA but others disagree on this point.

The General Medical Council (GMC) issued guidance on withholding and withdrawing life prolonging medical treatments in August 2002.[27] This will be discussed more fully in a later chapter of this book. Suffice it to say at this stage that the GMC guidance is thought by some to contravene the European Convention on Human Rights. There for the present the matter rests.

References.

1. Craig GM. Is sedation without hydration or nutrition in terminal care lawful? Medico Legal Journal 1994; **62**: 198-201.
2. Ashby M and Stoffell B. Artificial hydration and alimentation at the end of life: a reply to Craig. *Journal of Medical Ethics* 1995; **21**:135-140.
3. Fletcher GP. Prolonging life; some legal considerations. In Euthanasia and the Right to Death. Ed. Downing A. *Peter Owen*. London 1969.
4. Personal communication as from the Official Solicitor to the Supreme Court. Dec.16th 1994.
5. Macleod AD. The management of delirium in hospital practice. *European Journal of Palliative Care* 1997; **4**: 116-120.
6. Waller PC. Personal communication 12th January 1995.
7. Retired palliative medicine consultant. Personal communication 1997.
8. Principles of pain control in palliative care for adults. *Journal of the Royal College of Physicians of London* 2000; **34:** 350-352.
9. Harris G. 'Living on air' cult follower dies during holiday fast. *The Times* September 9th 1999 p3 cols 1-4.
10. Ethical decision making in palliative care. Artificial Hydration for people who are terminally ill. National Council for Hospice and Specialist Palliative Care Services. July 1997.
11. Huxtable R. Speaking at Conference on Euthanasia. Eastbourne, UK November 1999.

12. Price D. Euthanasia, pain relief and double effect. *Legal Studies* 1997; **17.2:** 323-342.

13. Euthanasia, Clinical Practice and the Law. Gormally L Ed. p50. *Linacre Centre London* 1994.

14. When doctors might kill their patients. a) Gillon R. Foreseeing is not necessarily the same as intending. *British Medical Journal* 1999; **318**:1431. b) Doyal L. The moral character of clinicians or the best interest of patients? Ibid. 1999; **318**: 1432-1433.

15. Austin Baker J. Personal communication, quoted with permission.

16. Lord Donaldson, quoted by Price. As ref.12 above.

17. Clarkson and Keating, quoted by Price. As ref.12 above.

18. The Queen and Her Majesty's Coroner for Inner London North ex parte Peter Francis Touche. Case No C/2000/2479. In the Supreme Court of Judicature Court of Appeal (Civil Division), March 21st 2001.

19. R v North Humberside ex parte Jamieson 1995 QBI, 25.

20. See ref 18 above at para 28.

21. Conclusions of Sir Thomas Bingham MR from ref 19 above, as 'distilled' by Mr I.Burnett QC and quoted by Lord Justice Brown in Touche. See ref 18 above at para 28.

22. Grove G.. Widower's battle to ease the loss of his perfect life. *The Times* January 19th 2002, p 5 cols 1-2.

23. McGhee v National Coal Board 1973 1WLR1. Comments by Lord Justice Simon Brown, quoted by him in Touche. See ref 18 above at para 20.

24. Ibid quoted by Brown S. in Touche. See ref 18 above at para 21.

25. Medical treatment at the end of life. A position statement. *Clinical Medicine* 2000; **1**:115-117.

26. Withholding and withdrawing life-prolonging medical treatment. Guidance for decision- making. British Medical Association. *BMJ Books* 1999.

27. Withholding and withdrawing life-prolonging treatments: good practice for decision-making. Guidance issued by the General Medical Council in August 2002.

Chapter 14

Guidelines Galore!

An overview by Gillian Craig

One of the positive outcomes of the hydration debate was the way palliative carers in the UK responded to my criticism. There was a lot of soul searching, and guidelines on the ethical use of artificial hydration in terminally ill people were thrashed out. I have yet to discover who commissioned the guidelines, but suspect that the Department of Health may have played a part. I was not party to the discussions.

1. The National Council for Hospice and Specialist Palliative Care Services (NCHSPCS) guidelines of 1997.

    i.) Artificial Hydration for people who are terminally ill.[1]
    ii). Cardiopulmonary Resuscitation (CPR) for people who are terminally ill.[2]
    iii). Changing Gear- guidelines for managing the last days of life in adults.[3]

Terminally ill people are defined by the NHS Executive as "…those with active and progressive disease for which curative treatment is not possible or not appropriate and from which death can reasonably be expected within 12 months." This definition was quoted by the NCHSPCS in the notes to their guidelines on CPR .

The first two guidelines on ethical decision-making in palliative care were published in July/August 1997. Both documents aimed to "rebut any charge of broadbrush therapeutic nihilism in hospice and specialist palliative care units in the UK".[4] The guidelines on the ethical use of artificial hydration for people are of crucial importance to the hydration debate, those on CPR less so. Both documents were published in the European Journal of Palliative Care with background information provided by Dunphy and Randall who chaired the committees that drafted the guidelines.[4] Laminated copies of the guidelines are available from the NCHSPCS of London, who hold the copyright. A full copy of the NCHSPCS guidelines on artificial hydration and CPR in terminally ill people, reprinted with the permission of the NCHSPCS, can be found in the Appendix at the back of this book.

Key points from the guidelines on artificial hydration…

- "A blanket policy of artificial hydration, or of no artificial hydration is ethically indefensible.
- Artificial hydration should be considered "…where dehydration results from a potentially reversible cause (e.g. overtreatment with diuretics and sedation, recurrent vomiting, diarrhoea and hypercalcaemia).
- When relatives express concern about lack of fluid or nutrient intake in dying patients "…Health care professionals may not subordinate the interests of patients to the anxieties of relatives but should nevertheless, strive to address those anxieties.

I first learnt that guidelines were imminent shortly before debating the issues with Dunphy at the Royal College of Physicians in June 1997. Dunphy unveiled the guidelines on artificial hydration during the debate. Later as we collected our slides from the projectionist he mentioned that the guidelines were to be published in the European Journal of Palliative Care in July. I obtained a copy by writing to the publishers, who kindly sent me the complete journal. It contained an article by Dunphy and Randall giving the background to the guidelines [4] - and so I discovered that the NCHSPCS guidance on the ethical use of artificial hydration had been produced in response to my critical paper in the Journal of Medical Ethics in 1994. Such is the secrecy of the powers that be, that no one mentioned this fact to me!

* * *

The discussion that follows includes extracts from an article by Killian Dunphy and Fiona Randall, as published in the European Journal of Palliative Care **4(4)**: 126-128, in 1997. © Hayward Medical Communications 1997. Extracts are quoted with permission and are printed in italics to set them apart from comments by Craig.

Dunphy and Randall explained how the guidelines evolved as follows-

"In September 1995, a working party drawn from the ethics committees of the Association for Palliative Medicine of Great Britain and Ireland and the National Council for Hospice and Specialist Palliative Care Services began work on two draft documents exploring the bases for ethical decision-making with respect to cardiopulmonary resuscitation (CPR) and artificial hydration (AH) in palliative care.

"The ethical problems posed by decisions either to implement or withhold/ withdraw such treatments in the context of palliative care have become increasingly evident in recent years. Some practitioners recognised that conflicting imperatives had the potential to cut to the core of 'hospice philosophy' and leave practitioners uncertain of the ethical defensibility of their practice. These documents were drafted with the intention of addressing those concerns." [4]

Consultation

"The membership of the joint working party was multiprofessional and the process of consultation has been wide-ranging. In preparing these documents we have taken advice from the British Medical Association, the Royal College of Nursing, the Department of Health and the National Health Service Executive. Specific advice on legal and ethical content has been provided by the Centre of Medical Ethics and Law, King's College, London.

"Useful comments and advice have also been received from many individuals, and the National Hospice Council has put the documents through a process of regional consultations. Almost two years into the process, and after eleven redrafts, the documents have been formally endorsed by the executive committee of the Association for Palliative Medicine and the National Council for Hospice and Specialist Palliative Care Services.

"Ultimately, the issues involved are emotive. Complete consensus will be hard to achieve. The success of such guidelines will rest on their congruence with established and evolving practice in disparate care settings (hospital, home, hospice, residential and nursing home) and their ability to unify differing approaches within a single framework that is internally consistent, intellectually defensible, emotionally appealing and intuitively correct." [4]

Artificial hydration

"In 1994, a paper was published in the Journal of Medical Ethics entitled 'On withholding nutrition and hydration in the terminally ill: has palliative medicine gone too far?' [5] *In it the author was robustly critical of what she saw as standard hospice practice in terms of its apparently unquestioning (and unquestionable) rejection of artificial hydration as a potential treatment option. The two years that have followed its publication have seen the paper become a focus for critical analysis of the clinical evidence presently available and for the crystallisation of arguments surrounding the ethical and legal dilemmas posed by the withholding or withdrawing of treatment in dying patients. The chief aim of these guidelines has been to encourage clinical teams providing palliative care to make patient-centred decisions, unhindered by the prejudice of an uncritical commitment to either an acute model of interventionist care or, indeed, to an overly rigid interpretation of hospice philosophy.*

"It seems reasonable to assert that the unilateral wholesale rejection of artificial hydration is as inappropriate in the care of individual patients as the assertion that all patients should have drips. Although staff will naturally afford a high level of importance to the concerns of relatives and the airing of such concerns will frequently be helpful in the formulation of shared decision-making, these views alone cannot be ethically determinative in management decisions. It is no more defensible to provide or omit a drip purely on the basis of the wishes of the relative than it is on the basis of the culture of the admitting unit or on the contents of its written philosophy. The issues of primary ethical or legal significance will be the wishes of the competent patient, the previously expressed competent wishes of the presently incompetent patient (concerning which relatives may provide valuable insights) and clinical judgements of 'best interest' (relating individual clinical assessment to research evidence and allowing evaluation of likely burdens and benefits of treatment)." [4]

Cardiopulmonary resuscitation

Dunphy and Randall explained the background to the CPR guidelines as follows-

"In 1991, the Health Service Commissioner in the UK upheld a complaint brought by the son of a 91-year-old lady who had not been informed of a decision that resuscitation should not be attempted on his mother following

her admission to hospital after a fall. The Commissioner was concerned at the lack of clear and agreed policies and guidelines in UK hospital trusts on appropriate consultation with relatives in such circumstances.

"As a result the government's Chief Medical Officer published a circular (PL/CMO (91) 22), making it clear that consultants carry ultimate responsibility for initiation, or otherwise, of CPR and that trusts should have policies in place providing guidance for junior medical and nursing staff." [4]

Informed consent and the obligation to discuss

These issues were discussed in some detail by Dunphy and Randall in connection with CPR, which I should explain to non-medical readers is the sort of resuscitation that takes place after a cardiac or respiratory arrest. The consensus view as stated in the NCHSPCS guidelines, is that the harms of CPR are likely to far outweigh the benefits in terminally ill patients. Dunphy and Randall noted that, *"There is no ethical obligation to discuss CPR with the majority of patients, for whom such treatment following assessment is likely to be futile. In the context of open and honest discussion, the raising of such issues may be redundant and potentially distressing."* [4]

If CPR is not discussed, Dunphy and Randall argue that failure to act in the event of a cardiac arrest may be ethically and legally defensible on the grounds of futility. However, they add the rider that *"omission on the basis of prolonging a poor quality of life almost certainly needs to rest on the patient's own assessment in order to be legally defensible."* [4] Moreover they comment *"Incompetent patients have had to be either insentient or enduring a life 'demonstrably intolerable to the patient' before courts in the UK have found it appropriate to omit or withdraw potentially life-sustaining treatment."* They then refer to the case of Airedale NHS Trust v Bland, and other less well known legal cases. The life-sustaining treatment in the case of Bland was of course artificial hydration and nutrition, not CPR, but Dunphy and Randall do not discuss this important legal point.

With respect to CPR they say that, *"...the concept of implied consent' on the basis that 'everyone knows you don't get resuscitated in a hospice' will not do for such patients. In agreeing to admission they are unlikely to have given their minds to this consideration and almost certainly cannot be said to have been 'adequately informed' on this specific issue...an open and honest exploration of the issues with those... who might benefit from attempts at resuscitation is justified (and perhaps ethically and legally required)."* [4] The same could be said about decisions to withhold artificial hydration from terminally ill patients!

* * *

Do not resuscitate orders as discussed above are relatively straightforward in principle, being advance decisions about whether or not to attempt CPR in the event of a cardiac or respiratory arrest. If these decisions are not made in advance responsibility for critical decisions about intervention may fall on a junior doctor who may be called to an emergency in the middle of the night. In the UK a government directive that came into operation in April 2001, requires that an advance decision about CPR be made on all hospital admissions, in consultation with the patient and appropriate relatives. However many doctors are reluctant to raise these sensitive matters for fear of frightening their patients. Many patients prefer to leave such matters to their doctor. Ideally CPR decisions should be made by a doctor who has full knowledge of the patient's clinical condition, and who understands the chances of successful resuscitation. Some patients would be incapable of giving informed consent if approached. Careful and sensitive discussion takes time and cannot be done quickly. Decisions made with care prevent inappropriate attempts to resuscitate hopelessly ill patients. Careful unrushed decisions are not always possible in the real world. Sometimes a brusque managerial approach takes over. Decisions can be influenced by factors such as ageism, finance, lack of resources, pressure on beds and so on. Although it may be appropriate to consult relatives if the patient is mentally incapacitated, relatives have no standing in law to intervene in medical decisions in the UK at present. However this may change if proxy health care decision makers are introduced in the future. Where a patient has made a valid advance directive that is applicable in the circumstances, their wishes should be respected.

In recent years the situation has become more complex, for "do not resuscitate" decisions have been interpreted in some quarters as "do not treat or prolong life in any way." (See for example the case of Mrs X, as outlined in chapter 6 of this book). Her problem came to the attention of the General Medical Council who now state categorically that- 'In holding discussions about CPR, you should make clear to the patient, the health care team and others consulted about the patient's care, that the provision of all other appropriate treatment and care would be unaffected by a decision not to attempt CPR.' [6]

The British Medical Association, Royal College of Nursing and Resuscitation Council joint statement on decisions relating to CPR of 2001.
Key points from a summary of basic principles.[7]

- Timely support for patients and people close to them, and effective, sensitive communication are essential.
- Decisions must be based on the individual patient's circumstances and reviewed regularly.
- Sensitive advance discussion should always be encouraged, but not forced.
- Information about CPR and the chances of a successful outcome needs to be realistic.
- Competent patients should be involved in discussion about attempting CPR unless they indicate that they do not want to be.
- Where people lack competence to participate, people close to them can be helpful in reflecting their views.
- *In an emergency,* if no advance directive has been made or is known, CPR should be attempted unless: the patient has refused CPR; the patient is clearly in the terminal phase of illness; or the burdens of treatment outweigh the benefits.[7]

Changing gear - managing the last days of life in adults

Had the hydration debate ended with publication of the guidelines on the ethical use of artificial hydration for people who are terminally ill, I could have returned home to a quiet retirement watering my plants. Sadly that did not prove possible, for no one who has a serious interest in medical ethics can afford to relax for long! All may seem quiet on the surface, while behind the scenes in committee rooms all over the world people are plotting the next move. Barely six months after publication of their guidelines on artificial hydration and CPR in the terminally ill, the NCHSPCS produced guidance on managing the last days of life in adults.

The guidelines entitled 'Changing Gear- guidelines for managing the last days of life in adults,' were published in a small booklet by the NCHSPCS in December 1997. This guidance was originally drafted by Dr Robert Dunlop for a NCHSPCS working party chaired by Dr Derek Doyle, and was later revised to conform to the Clinical Outcomes Group Guidelines by Professor Higginson, revision being financed by the National Health Service (NHS) Executive.[3]

The booklet 'Changing Gear...' sets out wide-ranging guidelines giving current thinking on the management of dying patients, as recommended by the NCHSPCS. They take a broad view, and provide much excellent advice, including sensitive comments about the needs of relatives. However the booklet dismisses the topic of dehydration in six lines that reflect the standard laissez-faire non-intervention approach beloved by traditional palliative carers [8,9]. As evidence of lack of benefit from intravenous or subcutaneous fluids in the last days of life, reference is made to the study by Ellershaw, Sutcliffe and Saunders of 1995 [8], which in my view is open to criticism [10]. The NCHSPCS list their guidance on the ethical use of artificial hydration in terminally ill patients with other references at the back of the booklet, but give no appropriate citation in the text.

Thus traditional old-school palliative care doctors, who feel threatened by those who consider hydration to be important, have done their best to regain ground, by closing their minds to views that do not support their case. Provided that the guidance in 'Changing Gear...' is used only for the final one or two days of life in a person who is irretrievably dying, little harm will be done. There is however a distinct danger that the earlier, more flexible guidelines on the ethical use of artificial hydration in patients who are terminally ill will be overlooked. If so we will be back at square one in the hydration debate.[5]

Experimental evidence of the benefits of hydration in the terminally ill and dying may be limited, but it is not negligible. One simply cannot ignore the work of Fainsinger and Bruera, the most accomplished workers in the field, for they have shown that delirium can be significantly reduced at the end of life if severe dehydration is avoided by the use of subcutaneous fluids. They concluded in 1997 that 'the data reported to date are insufficient to allow a final verdict on the benefit or harm of dehydration in terminally ill patients.' [11] So while the jury remains out we should all keep an open mind on the matter. Meanwhile, terminally ill patients who wish to receive subcutaneous fluids if they are dehydrated or at risk of becoming so, should make their wishes known.

2. General Medical Council guidance on 'Withholding and Withdrawing life prolonging treatments...'

A draft document was issued for consultation in May 2001, followed by a further draft issued by the Press Office in April 2002 for consideration by the Council in May 2002.[12] The current guidance was published in August 2002.[13]

The General Medical Council (GMC) guidance is very general in that it relates to decisions to withdraw or withhold life-prolonging treatment from patients with or without mental incapacity, if this is deemed to be in their best interest. Doctors are also permitted to withhold or withdraw artificial hydration and nutrition under some circumstances if the burden of provision appears to exceed the benefits. Early drafts contained relatively little about hydration, but in response to comments made during the consultation process the GMC convened a sub-committee to study this matter. The published guidance of August 2002 contained advice on the use of artificial hydration in patients who are imminently dying. Key sentences from paragraphs 81 and 26 read as follows:

Where death is imminent.

- *' Where death is imminent, in judging the benefits, burdens or risks, it usually would not be appropriate to start either artificial hydration or nutrition, although artificial hydration provided by less invasive measures may be appropriate where it is considered that this would be likely to provide symptomatic relief.* [12,13]
- *'Where death is imminent and artificial hydration and nutrition are already in use it may be appropriate to continue them if it is considered that the benefits outweigh the burdens to the patient.* [13] *(para 81)*
- *Patients who are dying should be afforded the same respect and standard of care as all other patients. Patients and their families and others close to them should be treated with understanding and compassion. (para.26).*

Where death is not imminent

The General Medical Council appear to have had considerable difficulty in reaching agreement about their guidance on withholding or withdrawing artificial hydration in patients in whom death is not imminent. Comparison of the final draft of May 2002 with guidance issued in August 2002 shows that subtle but significant changes in wording were made in the final months before publication. These indicate how rapidly opinion is shifting within the profession.

The draft of May 2002 stated-

*'Where death is not imminent it usually will be appropriate to provide artificial nutrition or hydration to meet the patient's assessed needs. **Exceptionally** (my emphasis), you may judge that a patient's condition is so severe that providing artificial nutrition or hydration may be of no benefit, or may cause suffering or be too burdensome to the patient in relation to the possible benefits. In these circumstances you must seek a second or expert opinion...'.*

Where death is not imminent: guidance of August 2002

The word 'exceptionally' does not appear in the published text. With the removal of this word the GMC give tacit recognition to the fact that decisions to withhold artificial hydration and nutrition from patients who are not imminently dying are not exceptional in clinical practice. It may seem strange to the general public that a professional organisation can be in some doubt about the frequency of this practice, but no one knows the answer to this question, for no records are kept.

Paragraph 81 of the text published in August 2002, contains the General Medical Council guidance on the provision of artificial nutrition or hydration in patients who are not imminently dying. Some such people depend on tube feeding or drips to sustain life, so decisions to withhold or withdraw tube feeding or drips can amount to a death sentence. The term "end of life decision-making" is used for these controversial and difficult decisions in medicine. The General Medical Council guidance in paragraph 81 was challenged recently in a judicial review. In his judgement of July 30th 2004 Mr Justice Munby ruled that the guidance was unlawful because it failed to recognise the heavy presumption in favour of life. The contentious guidance reads as follows:-

---

Where death is not imminent

'Where death is not imminent, it usually will be appropriate to provide artificial nutrition or hydration to meet the patient's assessed needs. However circumstances may arise where you judge that a patient's condition is so severe, and the prognosis so poor, that providing artificial nutrition or hydration may cause suffering or be too burdensome in relation to the possible benefits. In these circumstances as well as consulting the health care team and those close to the patient you must seek a second or expert opinion from a senior clinician (who might be from a second discipline such as nursing) who has experience of the patient's condition and who is not already directly involved in the patient's care. This will ensure that, in a decision of such sensitivity, the patient's interests have been thoroughly considered, and will provide necessary reassurance to those close to the patient and to the wider public.' [13]

The distinction between patients who are imminently dying and those who are not is an important one, but difficult to sustain in clinical practice. The GMC acknowledge this fact and note that *'It can be extremely difficult to estimate how long a patient will live, especially for patients with multiple underlying conditions. Expert help in this should be sought if you or the health care team are uncertain about a particular patient'.* [13]

This difficulty underlines the dangers of adopting a policy of non-intervention with respect to hydration in the last few days of life, as advocated by the National Council for Hospice and Specialist Palliative Care Services in their guidelines 'Changing Gear- Managing the Last Days of Life in Adults'. It would be infinitely preferable in my opinion, to try to maintain normal hydration in all patients who are dehydrated or at risk of becoming so, by offering them subcutaneous fluids or other measures as necessary, until death supervenes. If a patient is truly and irretrievably dying, such intervention will be needed on average for only 14 days. [11]

The need for a second opinion

The General Medical Council consultation document of May 2001 advised doctors to 'Always consult a clinician with relevant experience…when considering withdrawing artificial hydration and nutrition.' However later drafts and the final guidance of August 2002 distinguish between patients who are irrevocably and actively dying for example from terminal cancer, and other patients with potentially long-term survival. There now appears to be no requirement to obtain a second opinion with respect to such decisions in patients where death is imminent. However if death is not imminent a second or expert opinion from a senior clinician with experience of the patient's condition, and who is not already directly involved in the patient's care must be sought.

Thus the breadth of consultation has been extended to include the whole health care team and those close to the patient. This is good practice, not only to ensure that all voices are heard, but also to reduce the vulnerability of senior clinicians who are ultimately responsible for taking these difficult decisions. The suggestion that the crucial second opinion might come from a nurse should ring alarm bells, for it is an indication of the extent to which the medical profession are trying to distance themselves from these decisions and abdicate responsibility to others. The views of nurses and other health care workers who have been closely involved in the patient's care must of course be heard, but I am not convinced that it is necessarily wise to seek a second opinion of this crucial nature from people with no medical qualifications who have had no direct involvement in the patient's care.

In complying with the guidance proffered by the General Medical Council, the Council requires registered medical practitioners in the United Kingdom to 'take account of relevant guidance from professional bodies [14] and relevant protocols [7] within the health care setting in which you work'. Those who decide not to follow the GMC guidance, '…must be prepared to justify their actions and decisions to patients and their families, to colleagues and, where necessary, to the courts and the General Medical Council.' [15]

Conflict resolution

In the event of significant conflicts about the use of artificial hydration and nutrition, if the disagreement cannot be resolved after informal or independent review, the GMC recommend that legal advice should be sought. However there would be very little time in which to obtain this if the patient was close to death. Many NHS Hospitals and Trusts now have clinical ethics committees or other arrangements for access to clinical ethics support and advice. Where such arrangements are not available locally, advice of this kind can be obtained through the National Network of Clinical Ethics Committees based in Oxford [16]. It remains to be seen how effective this system will prove in an emergency. It must be recognised by all concerned that the value of an independent review will depend entirely on the wisdom, clinical judgement and humanity of those consulted. Sadly on present evidence, support for relatives who disapprove of the treatment given is hard to find.

The legal position

There is cause for concern about the legal position of doctors who withhold or withdraw life-sustaining medical treatment or sustenance. The General Medical Council were warned that their draft guidance issued in May 2002 appeared to be inconsistent with Article 2 of the European Convention on Human Rights. The Government of the UK signed the Council of Europe Agreement on the Protection of the Human Rights and Dignity of the Terminally Ill and Dying, which states- '... *the right to life- especially with regard to a terminally ill or dying person- is guaranteed by the member states, in accordance with Article 2 of the European Convention of Human Rights which states that "no-one shall be deprived of his life intentionally."* ' [17] (Sub-paragraph 9.c.iii)

Article 2, (para.14) of the Council of Europe document quoted above warns that '...*with regard to the terminally ill and dying...there is a grave danger that...justification may be sought under various pretences...to undermine the fundamental prohibition against taking life.*' [17]

The GMC guidance in August 2002 contained an appendix that summarised their understanding of key points of law.[18] The GMC noted that "...the Human Rights Act 1998 may have implications for this area of medical decision making...At present (English) case law confirms that existing common law principles are consistent with the European Convention on Human Rights." [19] "Not so!" - said Mr Justice Munby, a High Court Judge who considered the matter in a Judicial Review. His judgement was announced in the High Court on July 30th 2004.[20]

Key points from the High Court Judgement of July 2004

- The judgement states that "If life prolonging treatment is providing some benefit it should be provided unless the patient's life if thus prolonged, would from the patient's point of view be intolerable." [21] If there is any doubt about the matter it should be "resolved in favour of the preservation of life." [21]

- Paragraph 81 of the GMC guidance was declared unlawful as it failed to recognise "the heavy presumption in favour of life-prolonging treatment" [22] and failed to recognise that "it is for the competent patient, and not his doctor, to decide what treatment should or should not be given in order to achieve what the patient believes conduces to his dignity and in order to avoid what the patient would find distressing" [22]

- Decisions should be referred to court if there is a dispute between any of the medical professionals and relatives or carers as to whether artificial feeding should be withdrawn or withheld. [21,22]

- Artificial feeding could be withdrawn from a dying patient who lacked all awareness of what was happening.

The General Medical Council have appealed against the judgement. Meanwhile doctors in the UK are left in the bizarre situation that they are required to follow GMC guidance, but that guidance has been deemed unlawful!

164

3. Safe sedation practice

An intercollegiate working party was established at the request of the UK Academy of Medical Colleges to review the evidence on the safe provision of sedation services and produce recommendations applicable to the whole range of training and practice. Their report on 'Implementing and ensuring Safe Sedation Practice for healthcare procedures in adults' was published in November 2001.[23] The report addressed the use of short term sedation for procedures such as endoscopy and bronchoscopy, but had little or nothing specific to say about the use of sedation for days on end in a palliative care setting. However many comments made are of relevance to the use of sedation in palliative care. For example the report states that-

- 'Any drug which depresses the central nervous system has the potential to impair respiration, circulation or both.'
- ' Combinations of drugs especially sedatives and opioids should be employed with particular caution.'
- With combinations of drugs 'the safety margin between 'conscious sedation' and 'anaesthesia' can be reduced significantly.'
- If patients are deeply sedated to a point where they 'do not respond to verbal or physical stimuli, and may not maintain a clear airway…supervision requires the same level of training and skill'…as general anaesthesia.
- 'Sedatives and anxiolytics such as benzodiazepines have no analgesic properties when conventional doses are given systemically, and attempts to use them for pain control will result in significant overdose. Pain control requires the administration of a specific analgesic agent.'[23, 24]

The key point of the intercollegiate report was that safety will be optimised only if practitioners use defined methods of sedation for which they have received formal training. Various recommendations were made, one being that Royal Colleges, in association with the relevant sub-specialty organisations, should develop guidelines on sedation methods appropriate to clinical practice in their sphere of influence. It was also recommended that Royal Colleges and their faculties should incorporate the necessary instruction and assessment into training and revalidation programmes of those specialties that use sedation techniques. NHS Trusts should apply to sedation techniques the standard of the Clinical Negligence Scheme. Those responsible for commissioning and providing healthcare in the primary and private sectors should ensure that similar processes are in place to ensure a high standard of sedation practice.[23]

I would urge all doctors who use sedation in clinical practice to read this report and the recommendations in full. Copies are available from the Royal College of Anaesthetists in London. Attention was drawn to the report by a notice in the General Medical Council News of February 2002, so all doctors registered in the UK should be aware of its existence. Given that the General Medical Council consider that patients who are dying should be afforded the same respect and standard of care as all other patients, one can only hope that with the passage of time serious attention will be given to the safe use of sedation in palliative care.

In my view, whenever sedation is used, even in terminally ill patients, all reasonable precautions should be taken to ensure that the treatment does not hasten death. Potentially lethal dehydration should not be ignored unless the patient is irretrievably dying and death is imminent, or if the burden of treatment will clearly outweigh the benefits to the patient. However those who see death as a benefit take a rather different view, and use sedation without hydration quite freely at the end of life. This policy, dubbed 'terminal sedation', can be viewed as a subtle form of euthanasia. Concern about this remains at the heart of the hydration debate. It is crucial that palliative carers recognise the dangers of their ways, and take the message of the hydration debate to heart. Treatment regimes that will inevitably prove fatal should not be adopted, unless there is absolutely no other way of controlling unbearable symptoms at the end of life.

There are undoubtedly rare occasions when deep sedation or modern anaesthetic agents are required in palliative care to relieve distressing symptoms that cannot be controlled in any other way. Anaesthesia has been reported as a management option of last resort in delirium- for references see a review article on the management of delirium in hospital practice by Macleod.[25] However as Macleod observes, 'To anaesthetise in the absence of a life support system is generally considered to be unacceptable and a form of active euthanasia.' [25]

Artificial hydration given to prevent lethal dehydration can be regarded as a form of life support in a person who requires sedation for days on end. If doctors decide to withhold or withdraw such life support with intent to shorten life, they could be accused of committing euthanasia by omission, or 'passive euthanasia.' On the other hand if they decide to withhold or withdraw life-sustaining artificial hydration because the patient cannot tolerate it, or does not wish to have it, that is lawful. In the final analysis, if medical experts cannot agree, the legal profession may be required to decide whether treatment in an individual case was reasonable and lawful or not. In coming to a judgement lawyers should be mindful that 'Palliative care never has been, and never should be, an excuse for bad medicine'.[9]

4. Guidelines are not infallible

Some have clearly been written for the edification of the medical profession and the protection of patients, but others appear to have been devised for the protection of doctors who may be required to justify their actions in court. Guidelines drafted behind closed doors, by faceless committees, without due consultation should be viewed with deep suspicion. In this respect there are grounds for concern about guidance on pain control for palliative care in adults, issued by the Royal College of Physicians of London in 2000.[26] The guidance was prepared because the Department of Health and/or the euthanasia working party, chaired by Stephen Tumim, saw a need for clear guidelines on the use of opioids for pain relief in palliative care. The membership of the committee that drafted the guidance was not divulged, nor was the time scale of their deliberations. While much of the information given was basic and helpful to non-specialists, there were significant and serious omissions. For example no mention was made of the significant risk of dehydration during treatment with opioids (such as morphine) especially in the elderly. No mention was made of the use of subcutaneous fluids to maintain hydration when necessary. No reference was made to the NCHSPCS guidelines on the ethical use of artificial hydration in people who are terminally ill- instead their booklet 'Changing Gear- managing the last days of life in adults' was listed for further reading, although this guidance is clearly *not* appropriate for use at an earlier stage of an illness that could last for years. Continuous subcutaneous infusion of medication such as diamorphine, midazolam and methotrimeprazine was described as 'a very common method of controlling symptoms in the last hours or days of life…' No mention was made of the ethical problems raised by the use of sedation without hydration when continued for more than a few days. Thus the hydration debate was swept under the carpet. Objections were raised to no avail.

In the light of the Intercollegiate Working Party Report on Safe Sedation Practice [23] *sedation should not be promoted as a means of pain control in palliative care.*

5. Where are we now?

It is readily apparent that the medical profession is awash with guidance on the controversial subject of withholding and withdrawing life-prolonging medical treatment, including fluids and nutrition given by artificial, or assisted means. It is enough to turn the hair of any self-respecting medical practitioner grey!

The National Council (NCHSPCS) guidelines of July/August 1997 on the ethical use of artificial hydration in patients who are terminally ill were a brave attempt to answer my criticism and move the debate forward in a constructive way. Publication of the guidelines gave hope to those who put their trust in honest intellectual debate. Some progress was made and ground gained. When I attended the Palliative Care Congress in Warwick to debate the issues in 2000 I was assured on good authority that there are now very few hospices in the UK where the staff would be unable or unwilling to set up a drip should the need arise. That is good news for patients and relatives. In addition the emotional needs of relatives and friends are now receiving wider recognition. The General Medical Council guidance on the use of artificial hydration in the dying is helpful to some extent but will need to be revised in the light of the judicial review judgement of July 2004. Paragraph 81 of the GMC guidance has been deemed unlawful because it fails to recognise "the heavy presumption in favour of life-prolonging treatment." The patient's view as to whether their life is tolerable or intolerable should take precedence over the views of their doctor.

Some palliative carers are proving extremely resistant to change and seem reluctant to abandon the practice of sedation without hydration. A few still fly in the face of the evidence and deny that there is a problem. My call for a confidential enquiry into the use of parenteral sedation in palliative care in the UK has not been heeded, but data reported from other parts of the world indicates that its use is not unusual [27]. Sedatives such as midazolam and methotrimeprazine continue to be used quite freely to relieve or prevent distress in the dying. I hope for the sake of all concerned that the NCHSPCS guidelines of August 1997 on the ethical use of artificial hydration will be heeded.

In the USA some palliative carers remain unaware of the hydration debate as it has evolved in British journals. The Atlantic is still a significant dividing line where medical practice is concerned. In the USA 'managed death' by dehydration is seen as an alternative to physician-assisted suicide in some quarters, and 'Futile Care Theory' is all the rage. There is a danger that this approach could be imported to the UK unless wiser counsel prevails.

The life orientated approach to palliative care that I have proposed is in keeping with the best traditions of the hospice movement, and differs little from traditional palliative care as defined by the National Council for Hospice and Specialist Palliative Care Services in their evidence to the House of Lords Select Committee on Medical Ethics in 1993 [28]. The only major difference is recognition of the need to maintain hydration, if possible, to the end. Therefore the intensity of opposition to artificial hydration in some quarters seems quite extraordinary, for artificial hydration can be regarded as an essential physiological support system that may prevent many of the symptoms due to dehydration. It remains absolutely crucial to keep in mind the view that attention to hydration is not merely an option- it should be a basic part of good medicine and good palliative care.

All doctors who sedate their patients and withhold hydration without good reason would do well to consider an ancient Biblical saying-

**"A road may seem straightforward to one who is on it,
yet it may end as the way of death."** [29]

✱✱✱✱✱✱✱

Summary of progress made in the hydration debate in the UK in the last few years

Positive features

1. The medical profession has addressed the issue of hydration in terminally ill patients.
2. Guidelines on the ethical use of artificial hydration in terminally ill patients have been published and are available from the National Council for Hospice and Specialist Palliative Care Services in London.
3. A blanket policy of artificial hydration, or of no artificial hydration is ethically indefensible. Benefits and burdens of treatment must be carefully considered in every case.
4. The concerns of relatives and other carers about lack of fluid or nutritional intake must be addressed.
5. The general public are becoming aware of the ethical issues, and the legal profession have started to address the legal issues.
6. The General Medical Council acknowledge that patients who are dying should be afforded the same respect and standard of care as all other patients.
7. When death is not imminent, the need for an independent second opinion before withholding or withdrawing artificial hydration is now recognised.
8. A network of clinical ethics committees is evolving in the UK.

Other points of note

1. Palliative carers are proving reluctant to accept that artificial hydration may be needed in the last days of life.
2. The use of parenteral sedation in palliative care is not monitored or recorded.
3. The British Medical Association (BMA) and General Medical Council (GMC) approve the practice of withholding or withdrawing artificial hydration and / or nutrition from patients who are not dying under certain circumstances.
4. General Medical Council guidance applies to all practising doctors in the UK. Those who cannot comply for reasons of conscience should stand firm and be prepared to justify their action in court if need be.
5. The legal position remains unclear. There is concern that sedation without hydration is unlawful under some circumstances. Key elements of the GMC guidelines have been ruled unlawful.

References and notes

1. Ethical decision-making in palliative care. Artificial hydration for people who are terminally ill. *National Council for Hospice and Specialist Palliative Care Services*. London July/August 1997.

2. Ethical decision-making in palliative care. CPR for people who are terminally ill. *NCHSPCS* London July/August 1997. Laminated copies are available from NCHSPCS Fax 0207 723 5380.

3. Changing Gear- managing the last days of life in adults. *NCHSPCS*, London, December 1997.

4. Dunphy K, Randall F. Ethical decision making in palliative care. *European Journal of Palliative Care* 1997; **4**(4): 126-128. © Hayward Medical Communications, 1997.

5. Craig G M. On withholding nutrition and hydration in the terminally ill; has palliative medicine gone too far? *Journal of Medical Ethics*. 1994; **20**: 139-143.

6. Withholding and withdrawing Life-Prolonging Medical Treatments: Good Practice in Decision-making. *The General Medical Council*. August 2002. Para 91.

7. Decisions Relating to Cardiopulmonary Resuscitation: A joint statement by the British Medical Association, the Resuscitation Council (UK) and the Royal College of Nursing' BMA, London, February 2001. Available from all three bodies or browse on www.bma.org.uk. A summary was published in March 2001.

8. Ellershaw JE, Sutcliffe JM, Saunders CM. Dehydration and the dying patient. *Journal of pain and symptom management* 1995; **10**: 192-197.

9. Dunlop RJ, Ellershaw JE, Baines MJ, Sykes N and Saunders CM. On withholding nutrition and hydration in the terminally ill: has palliative medicine gone too far? A reply. *Journal of Medical Ethics* 1995; **21**:141-143.

10. For a critical review of reference 9 above see comments by Craig in chapter 4 of this book, No Water- No Life. Volume 1.

11. Fainsinger RL, Bruera E. When to treat dehydration in a terminally ill patient? *Support Care Cancer*, 1997: **5**(3): 205.

12. Withholding and withdrawing Life-Prolonging Treatments: Good Practice in Decision-making. The General Medical Council, London. Draft guidance of May 2002.

13. *The General Medical Council Guidance* of August 2002. Paragraph 81.

14. For example NHS Executive. 'Resuscitation Policy' HSC 2000/028. Department of Health, London, September 2000. Scottish Executive Health Department. 'Resuscitation Policy' HDL (2000) 22, Scottish Executive, November 2000.

15. As ref.13 at paragraph 95.

16. Contact ETHOX. Institute of Health Sciences, Old Road, Oxford OX3 7LF. Alternatively contact the Medical Ethics Alliance, UK. (www.medethics-alliance.org)

17. Council of Europe Agreement on the Protection of the Human Rights and Dignity of the Terminally Ill and Dying. Article 2 at sub-paragraph 9.c.iii and paragraph 14 as quoted to the General Medical Council by concerned Members of Parliament in 2003.

18. As reference 6 above. General Medical Council guidance of August 2002; Appendix A, p43-46, The legal background.
19. A National Health Trust v D (2000) 55 BMLR 19; NHS Trust A v M and NHS Trust B v H (2000) 58 BMLR 87. (As cited in General Medical Council guidance; August 2002: p46)
20. Queen's Bench Division, Regina (Burke) v General Medical Council before Mr. Justice Munby. Judgement July 30, 2004. Law Report. Incompatibility of GMC life-prolonging guidelines. *The Times*, (Tabloid version): p62, August 6th 2004.
21. Frean A. The new line separating life and death. *The Times* July 31st 2004, page 1 cols 1-4.
22. Rosenburg J. Dying man wins treatment fight. *The Daily Telegraph*, July31st 2004, page 1 and page 2, cols 1-4.
23. Implementing and ensuring Safe Sedation Practice for healthcare procedures in adults. Report of the Intercollegiate Working Party chaired by the Royal College of Anaesthetists. London November 2001. (See pages 6,7,10, 12)
24. Note. For a general article on pain control see Holdcroft A., Power I. Management of pain. British Medical Journal, 2003; **326**: 635-639.
25. Macleod AD, The management of delirium in hospital practice. *European Journal of Palliative Care*, 1997; **4(4)** : 116-120.
26. Principles of pain control in palliative care for adults. *Journal of the Royal College of Physicians of London*. 2000; **34**: 350-2.
27. Craig GM Terminal Sedation. *Catholic Medical Quarterly* Feb 2002. See chapter 8 of this book.
28. Key ethical issues in palliative care. Evidence to House of Lords' Select Committee on Medical Ethics. Occasional paper 3. *National Council for Hospice & Specialist Palliative Care Services*, London 1993.
29. The Bible, Proverbs, Chapter 16, verse 25.

Chronological Summary of Events

1990 Clash of cultures in a hospice provokes debate in the UK.

1991 Fainsinger and Bruera use subcutaneous fluids for symptom control.

1993 Law Lords allow Tony Bland to die.

1994 Fainsinger et al. Paper on subcutaneous fluids for rehydration in dying.

1994 Debate launched in Journal of Medical Ethics (JME).

1994 House of Lords Select Committee report on medical ethics.

1995 Debate continues in JME and Palliative Medicine.

        Working party set up to prepare guidelines in UK.

1996 Debate continues in the JME.

        Book by Randall & Downie on Palliative Care Ethics published.

1997 Issues debated at Royal College of Physicians of London. (RCP)

        National guidelines unveiled in London and published.

1998 Centre for Bioethics & Public Policy hold conference on palliative care.

        Medical Ethics and Law to be core subject in medical education.

        Euthanasia working party set up under auspices of RCP.

1999 The Times 'Back door euthanasia' report.

        RCP Conference on 'Ethical decisions at the end of life.'

        American Medical Association publish report on medical futility.

        British Medical Association publish controversial guidance.

2000 Pro-euthanasia activists support Boston Declaration on terminal sedation.

2001 Euthanasia working party and RCP endorse BMA guidance.

        Tumim Committee stress need for further debate by the profession & the public.

        Intercollegiate Working Party publish report on safe sedation practice.

2002 General Medical Council (GMC) guidance published.

2004 Patient challenges legality of GMC guidance in Judicial Review. Paragraph 81 of GMC guidance declared unlawful.

Epilogue

The changing face of palliative care.

The hydration debate as presented so far has been largely a discussion of the value of hydration in people dying of cancer. Yet such people represent only 24% of all deaths. The work of the hospice movement to date has concentrated mainly on cancer patients in whom pain control may be paramount. However in the UK and elsewhere the hospice movement is reaching out more and more to patients with illnesses such as AIDS, and motor neurone disease. When palliative care was accorded specialist standing in the UK in 1987, the agreed definition was 'the study and management of patients with active, progressive, far-advanced disease for whom the prognosis is limited and the focus of care is the quality of life'. Thus the scope of palliative care is considerable and the hospice approach could be extended to include patients with chronic illnesses such as strokes, dementia and arthritis. This trend is already apparent, and is viewed with considerable concern by some doctors. There is a danger that palliative carers may try to translate their experience with cancer patients to other patients who need a different approach. The special expertise of the hospice movement lies in pain control. Other groups of patients, such as those with strokes, dementia or various types of chronic arthritis, require different expertise that is best provided by doctors trained as geriatricians, psychogeriatricians or in some cases, rheumatologists. It is vital, for the sake of our patients that doctors continue to share their experience and discuss issues openly and honestly, with colleagues who may see things in a different light. Sectional warfare within the medical profession will not benefit the patient.

The hydration debate has shown that discussion is possible, although it can be a difficult and painful process for those involved. I hope and believe that our patients and their relatives will benefit in the long run. Medicine at its best involves the skilful use of art and science. The art of medicine involves creative listening, empathy, clinical intuition and wise judgement based on knowledge and professional experience. There must also be a willingness to use technological innovations when appropriate, and where available, for the benefit of the patient. No guidelines can translate this delicate process into a fool-proof course of action. They can only draw attention to essential aspects of the case that should be considered. Morality also comes into the equation, and so does the law, since this dictates the boundaries that must be respected by all citizens.

At the end of the day, the care of the dying, the terminally ill and the chronically disabled must be life-supportive, not death-orientated. There is a place for masterly inactivity in medicine, but masterly inactivity can merge into neglect. In the years that lie ahead, art and science must unite to decide what is appropriate in each case. There will inevitably be further debate and disagreement, but disagreement, rightly handled, leads to enlightenment and progress.

Appendix

National Council for Hospice and Specialist Palliative Care Services

ETHICAL DECISION-MAKING IN PALLIATIVE CARE:

Artificial Hydration for people who are terminally ill

This paper has been prepared by a Joint Working Party between the National Council for Hospice and Specialist Palliative Care Services and the Ethics Committee of the Association for Palliative Medicine of Great Britain and Ireland.

The paper is concerned with artificial hydration by nasogastric tube, gastrostomy, or subcutaneous or intravenous drip. It should be noted that good practice suggests decisions regarding artificial hydration should involve a multiprofessional team, the patient, and relatives and carers, but that the senior doctor has ultimate responsibility for the decision. However, a competent patient has the right to refuse artificial hydration, even if it may be considered of clinical benefit. Incompetent patients retain this right through a valid advance refusal.

1. A blanket policy of artificial hydration, or of no artificial hydration, is ethically indefensible.

2. Towards death, a person's desire for food and drink lessens. Study evidence is limited (see References) but suggests that artificial hydration in imminently dying patients influences neither survival nor symptom control. As such it may constitute an unnecessary intrusion.

3. Thirst or dry mouth in people who are terminally ill may frequently be caused by medication. In such circumstances artificial hydration is unlikely to alleviate the symptom. Good mouth care and reassessment of medication become the most appropriate interventions.

4. Appropriate palliative care will involve consideration of the option of artificial hydration, where dehydration results from a potentially correctable cause (e.g. over-treatment with diuretics and sedation, recurrent vomiting, diarrhoea and hypercalcaemia).

5. It is a responsibility of the clinical team to make assessments concerning the relevance of hydration to the experience of individual patients. The appropriateness of artificial hydration should be judged on a day-to-day basis, weighing up the potential harms and benefits. The practicalities of appropriate provision will vary according to setting, but good practice will require that patients needing artificial hydration are transferred to a unit equipped to provide such care.

6. Relatives at the bedside of dying patients frequently express concern about lack of fluid or nutrient intake. Health care professionals may not subordinate the interests of patients to the anxieties of relatives but should, nevertheless, strive to address those anxieties.

The appropriateness of artificial hydration continues to depend on regular assessment of the likely benefits and burdens of such intervention.

References

1. Oliver D. Terminal dehydration (letter). *Lancet* 1984: ii: 631.
2. Burge F. Dehydration symptoms of palliative care patients. *J Pain Symptom Manage* 1993:8: 454-64.
3. Ellershaw J.E, Sutcliffe J.M, Saunders C.M. Dehydration and the dying patient. *J Pain Symptom Manage* 1995 10(3): 192-197.
4. Craig G.M. On withholding nutrition and hydration in the terminally ill: has palliative medicine gone too far? *J Med Ethics* 1994: 20:139-43.
5. Regnard C, Mannix K. Reduced hydration or feeding in advanced disease — a flow diagram. *Palliative Medicine* 1991: 5: 161-64.
6. Dunphy K et al. Rehydration in palliative and terminal care: if not, why not? *Palliative Medicine* 1995: 9: 221-8.
7. Rosner F. Why nutrition should not be withheld from patients. *Chest* 1993: 104:1892-96.
8. Fainsinger R.L, MacEarchern T, Miller M.J et al. The use of hypodermoclysis for rehydration in terminally ill cancer patients. *J Pain Symptom Manage* 1994: 9: 298-302.
9. Billings J.A. Comfort measures for the terminally ill: is dehydration painful? *J Am Geriatr Soc* 1985: 33: 808- 10.
10. Printz L.A. Terminal dehydration: a compassionate treatment. *Arch Intern Med*
11. 1992: 152: 697-700.
12. Sommerville A. Cessation of treatment, non-resuscitation, aiding suicide and euthanasia. In: Fisher F, Macdonald N.J, Weston R. *Medical Ethics Today: its practice and its philosophy* London, BMJ Publishing Group, 1993: 165, 170-71.
13. Andrews M, Bell E.R, Smith S.A, Tischler J.F, Veglia J.M. Dehydration in terminally ill patients: is it appropriate palliative care? *Postgrad Med* 1993: 93: 201-08.
14. Tattersall M.H. Hypercalcaemia: historical perspectives and present management. *Support Cancer Care* 1993: 1: 19-25.
15. Twycross R.G, Lichter I. The terminal phase. In: Doyle D, Hanks G, MacDonald N. eds. *Oxford Textbook of Palliative Medicine,* Oxford, Oxford University Press, 1993:653-54.

National Council for Hospice and Specialist Palliative Care Services.
7 Floor. 1 Great Cumberland Place.
London WC1V 7PW
Tel 0207 723 1639 Fax 0207 723 5380
A Company limited by guarantee number 2044430
Registered Charity No 1005671
National Council for Hospice and Specialist Palliative Care Services

National Council for Hospice and Specialist Palliative Care Services

ETHICAL DECISION-MAKING IN PALLIATIVE CARE:

Cardiopulmonary Resuscitation (CPR) for people who are terminally ill

This paper has been prepared by a Joint Working Party between the National Council for Hospice and Specialist Palliative Care Services and the Ethics Committee of the Association for Palliative Medicine of Great Britain and Ireland.

Experience has shown that, when drawing up and implementing CPR policies, it is necessary to give particular consideration to the needs of terminally ill patients. It should be noted that good practice suggests that decisions regarding CPR should involve a multiprofessional team, the patient, and relatives and carers, but that the senior doctor has ultimate responsibility for the decision.

1. There is evidence [1,2,3] to suggest that, for terminally ill patients, the harms of CPR are likely far to outweigh the possible benefits. Evidence indicates that, almost invariably, CPR either fails to re-establish cardiopulmonary function, or succeeds only to result in further cardiopulmonary arrest with no intervening hospital discharge.

   (a) CPR is inappropriate if
      (i) there is virtually no chance of CPR re-establishing cardiopulmonary function; **or**
      (ii) successful resuscitation would probably result in a quality of life unacceptable to the patient (recognising that the focal point of any such decision would be the views of that patient); **or**
      (iii) it is contrary to the competent patient's expressed wishes.

   (b) CPR may be appropriate if
      (i) there is a reasonable chance of CPR re-establishing cardiopulmonary function; **and**
      (ii) successful resuscitation would probably result in a quality of life acceptable to the patient (recognising that the focal point of any such decision would be the views of that patient); **and**
      (iii) it is the competent patient's expressed wish. (See Point 5)

2. There is no ethical obligation to discuss CPR with the majority of palliative care patients, for whom such treatment, following assessment, is judged to be futile.[1-8] In the context of open and honest discussion, the raising of such issues may be redundant and potentially distressing.

3. If the likely outcome of a CPR intervention is uncertain, anticipatory decisions either to implement or withhold CPR should be sensitively explored with the patient. Both the likelihood of success and the resulting quality of life will be appropriate issues for discussion. Review of any such decision may be appropriate with change in the patient's clinical situation.

4. Should a patient be likely to benefit from CPR and would wish for it, the extent of CPR facilities and expertise available in any admitting unit ought to be discussed with the patient, ideally prior to admission. Limited

availability of such facilities in specialist palliative care units need not undermine appropriateness of admission in early disease as patients may accept such admission on the understanding that initial resuscitative measures will be instituted and transfer to a unit equipped to undertake CPR will be arranged in the event of a cardiac arrest actually occurring.

5. Consideration should be given to CPR policy early in the involvement of the clinical team. In the absence of an anticipatory decision or a valid advance refusal, at the time of cardiorespiratory arrest, the patient is by definition incompetent to make a decision regarding CPR and therefore it is the doctor's legal responsibility to act in the patient's best interests.

Notes

(I)   'Terminally ill people are those with active and progressive disease for which curative treatment is not possible or not appropriate and from which death can reasonably be expected within twelve months." (from *Care of People with Terminal Illness,* NAHAT, 1991; EL (95) 22, NHS Executive 23 February 1995; and *Specialist Palliative Care: A Statement of Definitions,* NCHSPCS, 1995).

(II)   Decisions concerning CPR policy for individual patients should be clearly recorded and communicated to all relevant staff, including deputising or GP cooperative services.

(III)   It would be helpful if ambulance service providers could be made aware of the policy relating to individual patients who would not benefit from, or wish for, CPR. Local mechanisms for the communication of anticipatory decisions to paramedical staff in relation to individual patients in the domiciliary setting would also be helpful.

References

1. Dautzenberg P.L.J, Broekman T.C.J, Hooyer C, Schonwetter R.S, Duursma S.A. Review: Patient-related predictors of cardiopulmonary resuscitation of hospitalised patients, *Age and Aging* 1993: 22: 464.475.

2. Bedell S.E, Delbanco T.L, Cook E.F, Epstein F.H. Survival after cardiopulmonary resuscitation in the hospital, *N Engl J Med* 1983: 309: 569-575.

3. Ebell M.H. Pre-arrest predictors of survival following in-hospital cardiopulmonary resuscitation; comparison of two predictive instruments, *Resuscitation* 1994: 28: 2 1-25.

4. British Medical Association and Royal College of Nursing. *Decisions relating to cardiopulmonary resuscitation.* Joint statement in association with the Resuscitation Council (UK), BMA House, London, March 1993.

5. Sommerville A. Cessation of treatment, non-resuscitation, aiding suicide and euthanasia. In: Fisher F. *Medical Ethics Today: Its practice and philosophy,* London BMJ Publishing Group, 1993: 173.

6. Murphy D.J, Burrows D, Santilli S et al. The influence of the probability of survival on patients preferences regarding cardiopulmonary resuscitation, *N Engl J Med* 1994: 330: 545-549.

7. Miller D.L, Gorbien M.J, Simbartl L.A, Jahnigen D.W. Factors influencing physicians in recommending in-hospital cardiopulmonary resuscitation, *Arch Intern Med* 1993:153:1999-2003.

8. George A.L, Folk B.P, Crecelius P.L, Campbell W.B. Pre-arrest morbidity and other correlates of survival after in-hospital cardiopulmonary arrest, *Am i Med* 1989: 87: 28-34.

Joint Working Party between The National Council for Hospice and Specialist Palliative Case Services and the Ethics Committee of the Association for Palliative Medicine of Great Britain and Ireland

Mrs B Biswas, Matron, LOROS, Leicestershire Hospice, Leicester
Dr K Dunphy, Macmillan Consultant in Palliative Medicine, Macmillan Runcie Day Hospice, St Albans.
Dr J Ellershaw, Medical Director, Marie Curie Centre, Liverpool
Dr M Minton, Consultant in Palliative Medicine, Sir Michael Sobell House Palliative Care Unit, The Oxford Radcliffe Hospital
Mr D Oliviere, Macmillan Lecturer in Social Work and Palliative Care, School of Social Work and Health Sciences, Middlesex University, Enfield
Mr D Praill, Chief Executive, Help the Hospices, London
Dr F Randall, Consultant in Palliative Medicine, Macmillan Unit, Christchurch Hospital, Dorset
Dr G Rathbone, Consultant in Palliative Medicine, LOROS, Leicestershire Hospice, Leicester
Dr T Tate, Consultant in Palliative Medicine, The Margaret Centre, Whipps Cross Hospital; Consultant in Palliative Medicine, St Bartholomew's Hospital, London

National Council for Hospice and Specialist Palliative Care Services,
7th Floor, 1 Great Cumberland Place,
London WC1V 7PW
Tel: 0207 723 1639 Fax 0207 723 5380
A Company limited by guarantee number 2644430
Registered Charity No 1005671

A final thought

Looking back on a decade of debate and struggle to get my colleagues in palliative medicine to abandon the use of sedation without hydration, I sometimes feel that little ground has been gained. Yet slowly, slowly, the truth is dawning. And so it seems appropriate to end this book with a poem of hope and promise. By a strange coincidence the poem I have chosen was written by Arthur Hugh Clough- the same man who wrote those words beloved by the medical profession: "Thou shalt not kill; but need'st not strive officiously to keep alive."

Say Not The Struggle Nought Availeth

Say not the struggle nought availeth,
The labour and the wounds are vain,
The enemy faints not, nor faileth,
And as things have been, they remain...

If hopes were dupes, fears may be liars,
It may be, in yon smoke concealed,
Your comrades chase, e'en now, the fliers,
And but for you, possess the field.

For while the tired waves, vainly breaking,
Seem here no painful inch to gain,
Far back, through creeks, and inlets making,
Comes silent, flooding in, the main.

And not by eastern windows only,
When daylight comes, comes in the light;
In front, the sun climbs slow, how slowly,
But westward, look, the land is bright.

(Arthur Hugh Clough. 1819-1861)

Bibliography

Cameron N (Ed). Death without Dignity. Euthanasia in Perspective. Rutherford House Books. Edinburgh 1990.

Clark D, Hockley J, Ahmedzai S, (Ed). New Themes in Palliative Care. Open University Press 1997.

Curran C. Politics, Medicine and Christian Ethics. Fortress Press Philadelphia 1973.

Euthanasia, Clinical Practice and the Law. Ed. Gormally L. The Linacre Centre, London 1994.

Euthanasia. A Christian perspective. Ed. Brown H, Gibbs K. The Church of Scotland Board of Social Responsibility. Publisher Saint Andrew Press. Edinburgh. 1995.

Euthanasia examined: Ethical, Clinical and Legal Perspectives. Ed. Keown J. Cambridge University Press 1995.

Habgood J. Being a Person. Hodder and Stoughton, London 1998.

Hoefler J.M. Managing Death. Westview Press 1997.

Oderberg D. Applied Ethics. Blackwell. 2000.

Randall F and Downie R.S. Palliative Care Ethics. Oxford University Press 1996.

Ramsay D.J. and Booth D.A. (Ed). Thirst. Physiological and Psychological Aspects. Springer-Verlag London 1991.

Ramsay P. The Patient as a Person. Explorations in Medical Ethics. Yale University Press. New Haven 1970.

Siegal B. Love, Medicine and Miracles. Arrow 1988.

Smith Wesley J. "Forced Exit". Spence Publishing, Dallas, Texas. Revised edition 2003.

Vanier J. Our Journey Home. Hodder and Stoughton London 1997.

Wyatt J. Matters of Life and Death. Inter-Varsity Press. Leicester 1998.

Index